REPRODUCTIVE TECHNOLOGIES

Other Books in the Current Controversies Series:

REPRODUCTIVE TECHNOLOGIES

David Bender, *Publisher*
Bruno Leone, *Executive Editor*

Scott Barbour, *Managing Editor*
Brenda Stalcup, *Senior Editor*

Carol Wekesser, *Book Editor*

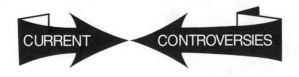

Cover photo: Jim Olive/Peter Arnold, Inc.

Library of Congress Cataloging-in-Publication Data

Reproductive technologies / Carol Wekesser, book editor.
      p. cm. — (Current controversies)
    Includes bibliographical references and index.
    ISBN 1-56510-376-9 (pbk. : alk. paper). — ISBN 1-56510-377-7
(lib. bdg. : alk. paper)
    1. Human reproductive technology—Social aspects. 2. Human reproductive technology—Moral and ethical aspects. I. Wekesser, Carol, 1963-   . II. Series.
RG133.5.R467   1996
176—dc20   95-35484
                                              CIP

Contents

Chapter 2: Should Postmenopausal Women Become Pregnant?

Yes: Pregnancy After Menopause Is Acceptable

No: Women Should Not Become Pregnant After Menopause

Chapter 3: Is Surrogate Motherhood Beneficial or Harmful?

Chapter 4: Do Reproductive Technologies Result in the Unethical Treatment of Embryos?

Yes: Reproductive Technologies Result in the Unethical Treatment of Embryos

No: Reproductive Technologies May Not Result in the Unethical Treatment of Embryos

Chapter 5: What Would Be the Effect of Regulating Reproductive Technologies?

Regulating Reproductive Technologies Would Be Beneficial

Regulating Reproductive Technologies Could Be Harmful

Foreword

By definition, controversies are "discussions of questions in which opposing opinions clash" (Webster's Twentieth Century Dictionary Unabridged). Few would deny that controversies are a pervasive part of the human condition and exist on virtually every level of human enterprise. Controversies transpire between individuals and among groups, within nations and between nations. Controversies supply the grist necessary for progress by providing challenges and challengers to the status quo. They also create atmospheres where strife and warfare can flourish. A world without controversies would be a peaceful world; but it also would be, by and large, static and prosaic.

The Series' Purpose

The purpose of the Current Controversies series is to explore many of the social, political, and economic controversies dominating the national and international scenes today. Titles selected for inclusion in the series are highly focused and specific. For example, from the larger category of criminal justice, Current Controversies deals with specific topics such as police brutality, gun control, white collar crime, and others. The debates in Current Controversies also are presented in a useful, timeless fashion. Articles and book excerpts included in each title are selected if they contribute valuable, long-range ideas to the overall debate. And wherever possible, current information is enhanced with historical documents and other relevant materials. Thus, while individual titles are current in focus, every effort is made to ensure that they will not become quickly outdated. Books in the Current Controversies series will remain important resources for librarians, teachers, and students for many years.

In addition to keeping the titles focused and specific, great care is taken in the editorial format of each book in the series. Book introductions and chapter prefaces are offered to provide background material for readers. Chapters are organized around several key questions that are answered with diverse opinions representing all points on the political spectrum. Materials in each chapter include opinions in which authors clearly disagree as well as alternative opinions in which authors may agree on a broader issue but disagree on the possible solutions. In this way, the content of each volume in Current Controversies mirrors the mosaic of opinions encountered in society. Readers will quickly realize that there are many viable answers to these complex issues. By questioning each author's conclusions, students and casual readers can begin to develop the critical thinking skills so important to evaluating opinionated material.

Current Controversies is also ideal for controlled research. Each anthology in the series is composed of primary sources taken from a wide gamut of informational categories including periodicals, newspapers, books, United States and foreign government documents, and the publications of private and public organizations. Readers will find factual support for reports, debates, and research papers covering all areas of important issues. In addition, an annotated table of contents, an index, a book and periodical bibliography, and a list of organizations to contact are included in each book to expedite further research.

Perhaps more than ever before in history, people are confronted with diverse and contradictory information. During the Persian Gulf War, for example, the public was not only treated to minute-to-minute coverage of the war, it was also inundated with critiques of the coverage and countless analyses of the factors motivating U.S. involvement. Being able to sort through the plethora of opinions accompanying today's major issues, and to draw one's own conclusions, can be a complicated and frustrating struggle. It is the editors' hope that Current Controversies will help readers with this struggle.

"Reproductive technologies . . . are allowing hundreds of families each year to have babies. But the miraculous new techniques have raised troubling questions about medical science's increasing ability to tinker with biological processes."

Introduction

Infertility is an age-old problem. Even the Old Testament of the Bible recounts a couple's struggle with infertility in the story of Abraham and Sarah, a couple who yearned for a child. After years of childlessness, Abraham and Sarah resorted to a "surrogate mother" of a sort when Abraham took a concubine and had a son, Ishmael; later, they had their own biological son, Isaac.

Many childless people have experienced the same disappointment and desperation Abraham and Sarah felt. About 8.5 percent of U.S. married couples are infertile. Until recently, infertile couples either adopted other people's children or accepted their childless state and found other ways of leading fulfilling lives. But while these alternatives could ultimately be satisfying, the fact remained that for many people childlessness was a frustrating, heart-wrenching situation.

In recent decades those wanting children have had another alternative: reproductive technologies. "Reproductive technologies" refers to a wide range of procedures. Artificial insemination, in which sperm is artificially introduced into the uterus, has been used for years and is probably the simplest of the reproductive technologies. In vitro fertilization, pioneered in 1978, involves fertilizing an egg with sperm in a petri dish, then transferring the embryo into the woman's uterus for gestation.

Some of the more recent technologies are spin-offs of in vitro fertilization: ZIFT, or zygote intrafallopian transfer, entails putting the embryo into one of the woman's two fallopian tubes (tubes that conduct the egg from the ovary to the uterus) and then allowing it to travel to and implant in the woman's uterus. GIFT, or gamete intrafallopian transfer, involves placing the sperm and the unfertilized egg into the fallopian tubes, which is followed by conception and implantation in the uterus. With zona cracking or drilling, scientists can now even cut the outside of an egg and insert a single sperm, thereby causing fertilization. The embryo is then implanted in the woman.

Which technology someone chooses largely depends on the cause of their infertility. For example, women with blocked fallopian tubes may utilize in vitro fertilization to become pregnant. Men with few or weak sperm may benefit from GIFT, ZIFT, or zona drilling. Women who want to experience pregnancy, childbirth, and parenting without the involvement of a man may choose to become artificially inseminated with sperm from a donor. Similarly, a man who wishes to be a father without being a husband may find a surrogate to be artificially inseminated and to bear a child.

Reproductive technologies promise to answer the prayers of many people who want children. They offer hope to those unable or unwilling to adopt and to those who want a newborn child that is genetically related to at least one of the parents. "I feel fortunate that I live in a society where the medical profession may be able to make it possible for me to have a baby," said one woman who used in vitro fertilization.

But to others the potentially negative medical, social, and economic consequences of reproductive technologies are reason enough to ban or strictly regulate these new procedures. The possible social ramifications of reproductive technologies are perhaps the most disconcerting to many people. Theoretically, a child conceived through reproductive technology could have five parents: a sperm donor biological father, an egg donor biological mother, a gestational surrogate mother who would carry and give birth to the baby, and a social mother and father—the couple that would care for and raise the child. While this situation may be rare, the relationships involved in cases of reproductive technology can be complex. The emotional consequences to the child and the adults involved are unknown, as are the consequences to society as a whole. As sociologist John Edwards writes in the *Journal of Marriage and the Family*, "The new reproductive technologies signal the obsolescence of marriage and the family. . . . Implicitly the innovations suggest that the family of the future may merely consist of one socialized adult and an offspring."

Mark Nichols, a writer for *Maclean's,* states that "reproductive technologies . . . are allowing hundreds of families each year to have babies. But the miraculous new techniques have raised troubling questions about medical science's increasing ability to tinker with biological processes." *Reproductive Technologies: Current Controversies* examines these troubling questions by presenting the differing views of the patients and physicians involved in these new medical procedures and of the feminists and social critics concerned with the consequences of such practices.

Chapter 1

Are Reproductive Technologies Beneficial or Harmful?

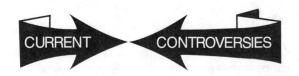

Reproductive Technologies: An Overview

by Margery Stein

About the author: *Margery Stein is a freelance writer based in New York City. She frequently writes on social issues.*

Ever since he was about 5, Bill Cordray had been haunted by a peculiar thought: *I am not my father's son.* "I felt connected to my mother, but not at all to my dad. I loved him, but he was distant to me, and we were different in about every way: our looks, our personalities, our interests."

Soon a fantasy took root in the young Cordray's mind. "I decided that I was the product of an affair," he says, "but I was deeply ashamed of those thoughts so I didn't confront my mother."

It took a major trauma—the death of his younger brother, Dick, when Cordray was 37—to bring the facts to light. "My dad had died the year before," Cordray, now a 49-year-old architect, remembers. "After Dick's funeral, my mom and I were talking about him and about my dad, and I said, half-jokingly, 'You know, I used to think Dad wasn't really my father.'" Abruptly, his mother blurted out the long-suppressed truth. "Well, since you do suspect," she said, "he really *wasn't* your father."

Cordray's "dad," the term he uses to distinguish the man who raised him from his biological parent, was infertile, and his mother had turned to donor insemination (the use of sperm from a donor other than the husband). The news was a shock to Cordray but also a great relief. "It cleared up the mystery I'd been living with all my life."

Cordray's mother knew nothing about his biological father beyond the fact that the man had been a medical student, class of '45. "Her doctor had told her it wasn't important to have much information about the donor," says Cordray, who was determined to track down this mystery man. "I wasn't trying to replace my dad," he says, "or get money from this person, or even develop a close relationship. I just wanted to know where I came from."

He began by calling the clinic where his mother had been inseminated. It was still in business, but his records were long gone. Finally he came up with the medical school's 1945 class list and painstakingly began to weed out names. He began to suspect that the donor might have been his mother's doctor. "She told me he'd made a special trip to the clinic the day she was there, to bring in the semen samples," Cordray recalls. "Back then, because of a lack of donors, doctors often used their own semen."

The doctor was retired and living nearby—yet six years passed before Cordray could summon the nerve to meet with him. Eventually, he did approach the doctor while the man was gardening in his yard. "I told him about the insemination and asked if he could help me get information about my father," Cordray says. "He couldn't talk to me then, and I later found out he'd been in an auto accident and had suffered extreme memory loss. We talked a few more times, but to no avail."

Cordray now believes that another physician, who was a partner in the clinic, is actually his birth father, "but I can't be sure unless I get a DNA check." That isn't likely to happen. "We've met, but he's 87 and senile, so he can't express much to me."

Now, Cordray says, the issue has shifted from finding his father to changing the practice of secrecy surrounding donor insemination (DI) cases. He has met other DI adoptees (the name they call themselves), and, he says, "We're primarily concerned with convincing DI parents that they should know more about the donors, and at least have access to their medical records. We want children to have the right to know who their biological father is."

Sperm Bank Secrecy

Artificial insemination has been shrouded in secrecy for more than a century, ever since men began donating sperm to help childless couples conceive. Physicians routinely kept couples and donors in the dark about each other and counseled parents-to-be not to tell their offspring about their origins. Even when the first sperm bank opened its doors at the University of Iowa in 1950, the tradition of secrecy endured. "The cover-up was based on the belief that the husband's ego couldn't tolerate the pain of infertility," says Patricia Mahlstedt a Houston psychologist who has studied donor secrecy.

"Prospective parents now want access to [sperm] donors' medical records."

Recently, a small but vocal minority of DI adoptees has been challenging the tradition of closed records. Fueling the debate are the recognition of the importance of genetic information and the insidious effect of secrecy on families, plus a policy of openness in the more recent practice of egg donation.

As a result, a change of attitude is under way. Some sperm-bank officials say prospective parents now want access to donors' medical records and are more concerned about the rights of their child-to-be. The American Fertility Society (AFS), one of the main industry associations, has amended its guidelines from advising anonymity to stating that secrecy may or may not be beneficial. Although only a few sperm banks are as yet willing to release donors' names, according to Barbara Raboy, executive director of the progressive Sperm Bank of California in Oakland, just under half of all their donors have agreed to allow DI offspring access to their biological father's name when the children turn 18.

> *"Only a few sperm banks are as yet willing to release donors' names."*

"The important thing for a child is to be able to visualize the donor," says Annette Baran, a specialist in infertility and co-author of the book *Lethal Secrets: The Psychology of Donor Insemination* (Amistad Press). "It's not a teaspoon of sperm, it's a *person*."

Leslie and Paul are one DI couple who agree. Both 38, they first went to the Oakland Sperm Bank nine years ago, after learning that Paul was infertile. Today they have three sons, all from the same donor. "He has agreed to let the kids see him when they're 18," says Leslie. "We've already told them."

"I felt it was important that they know," says Paul, "because if they found out in some other way, they'd wonder what else we'd told them that wasn't true."

Record-Keeping Problems

No one can say how large the DI population is. A survey released by the Office of Technology Assessment in 1987 found that about 30,000 babies were born in the United States in 1986–87 through the gift of a stranger's sperm. According to one estimate, there could be 1,000,000 DI adults in this country today.

In an industry in which regulations are few, record keeping can be less than accurate. The AFS and the American Association of Tissue Banks (AATB) issue voluntary guidelines on record keeping and other sperm-bank procedures, but these organizations have no real teeth. Only New York State, with the strictest licensing requirements in the United States, mandates that insemination results be reported back to the sperm banks.

No one can even be certain how many such banks exist. "By our count there are 135," says John Critser, chairman of AATB's reproductive council. "But according to one recent estimate, there may be as many as 1,100, including hundreds of small-scale operations."

There is also a lack of reliable data on the number of live births per donor. "We have no authority to require physicians to communicate with us," says Critser, "and in general, they don't. So few banks have any comprehensive data on pregnancies."

Many of the programs accept fewer than 10 percent of donors who volunteer, and this shortage of good donors (those with a solid health background and a high sperm count) can also lead to abuses of the system. Mike, a 35-year-old engineer who has been donating sperm once or twice a week for 15 years, says that his clinic claims he has fathered more than 400 offspring. "I thought that was an enormous number," he says, "but they told me it was low for a popular donor—that others have produced over 1,000 children."

Those numbers are worrisome because the risk of unwitting incest, while small, does exist. "Doctors have twice stopped marriages between children conceived with sperm from the same donor," says Lori Andrews, a law professor specializing in reproductive technologies at Chicago-Kent College of Law.

Picking a donor is, in effect, an exercise in baby design. The prospective parent flips through sperm-bank catalogs, which list statistics such as height and hair color for 100 or more number-coded males. If a thumbnail sketch interests a customer, she requests the lengthier, more detailed personal and medical history.

Some banks have become quite creative about their facts on file. Cryogenic Laboratories, Inc., in Roseville, Minnesota, has developed a unique computerized system called DADS (data-assisted donor selection) that is available to physicians. If your doctor has DADS, you can use this software to select a donor based on your desired characteristics and compare data on several donors.

The Fertility Clinics

Donor insemination is a low-tech procedure compared to the newer, more sophisticated reproductive technologies, including egg donation, that were pioneered in 1978 when Britain's Baby Louise became the first "test-tube baby" born via in-vitro fertilization (IVF, fertilizing either a donor egg or the mother's own egg in the laboratory).

Since the United States made its own IVF breakthrough in 1981 with the birth of Baby Elizabeth, the infertility business has ballooned into an estimated $2-billion-a-year industry, with some 300 fertility clinics nationwide performing in-vitro fertilization and related technologies. Physicians claim success rates for the various treatments of 15 to 20 percent, but those rates drop dramatically when the recipient is over 35, notes Andrea Braverman, Ph.D., director of psychological services at Pennsylvania Reproductive Associates in Philadelphia.

IVF is generally considered one of the most effective treatments for male fertility problems, which are responsible for 30 to 40 percent of failures to conceive. But since IVF does not work for many men with severe sperm abnormalities, embryologists have developed a series of ever-more-precise "micromanipulation" techniques

"Egg donation can be stressful and potentially hazardous."

aimed at coaxing sluggish or malformed sperm to pierce the egg.

First came partial zona dissection, which involves making a small opening in the egg's outer membrane to help sperm swim inside. Next was subzonal insertion, in which a tiny needle is used to puncture that membrane and shoot multiple sperm into the egg. The latest development, intracytoplasmic sperm injection (ICSI), entails shooting a single sperm into the egg. "This is our best hope of giving men with minimal sperm quality a chance at impregnating their spouses," says Dr. Arthur Wisot, staff physician at the Center for Advanced Reproductive Care in Redondo Beach, California, and co-author of *New Options for Fertility* (Pharos Books).

> *"The testing of genes might be just one short step from manipulating them."*

Within the past couple of years, an increasing number of clinics have begun performing ICSI in conjunction with "assisted hatching," a procedure that "helps the embryos become attached to the uterine lining," says Jacques Cohen, Ph.D., scientific director of assisted reproduction at Cornell University Medical College in New York City. "It appears to improve the success rate in the most difficult patients," he says.

A Complicated Science

With an estimated 2.3 million married couples considered infertile (unable to conceive after trying for a year or more), the potential market for services is huge. In practice, however, only a privileged minority can afford to pay fees that range from $8,000 to $15,000 for a single attempt with donor eggs. (The donor receives between $1,500 and $2,000.) These costs are much higher than those for artificial insemination, which run about $300 per attempt.

The time commitment is substantial as well: From start to finish, an IVF procedure takes about four weeks. The standard procedure is as follows: The egg donor receives medication for 7 to 12 days to stimulate egg production. When she starts to ovulate, the eggs are retrieved by a needle inserted through the vaginal wall; they are then united with sperm in a petri dish. A few days later, the fertilized eggs are implanted in the prospective mother's womb.

There are also two alternate implantation procedures: gamete intrafallopian transfer, in which eggs and sperm are placed directly into the fallopian tubes, and zygote intrafallopian transfer, in which sperm and eggs are fertilized in vitro, then inserted into the fallopian tubes.

Unlike sperm donation, a simple collection procedure, egg donation can be stressful and potentially hazardous. "In rare instances, overstimulating the ovaries can be life threatening," says Dr. Wisot. "There's also the risk of the needle's hurting something else in the body."

As for legal protection, egg donors are in a kind of no-woman's-land. "The law is not well developed with respect to parental rights and responsibilities," says Lori Andrews. "Only two states, Oklahoma and Florida, have laws saying egg recipients are the legal parents."

With so many potential problems, women are hardly lining up to give away their eggs. Still, the experience has its rewards. Sue Scott, 37, herself the mother of two, began donating eggs for IVF when she was 29, on condition that she meet the recipient couples and the offspring. "I don't feel these children are mine, but I need to know they're O.K.," she says. Scott's eggs produced five children, and she stopped donating at 35, the typical cutoff age for women (sperm donors may remain active longer). "I'm in touch with all five kids," she says, "and I get Christmas and birthday pictures. I made these people happy. It's a really terrific feeling."

The Brave New World

At the crossroads where reproductive technology and genetic forecasting meet, stunning developments are taking place. Work is already under way to alter the DNA of pre-embryos with genetic defects. Using a glass needle thinner than a human hair, scientists at East Virginia Medical School in Norfolk withdrew a single cell from a pre-embryo (a fertilized egg) in a test tube and analyzed its DNA for the deadly Tay-Sachs disease. After altering the defective gene they implanted the pre-embryo in the mother's uterus. Result: a healthy baby girl.

Other tests certain to set off alarms will be coming on line soon. "There will be tests on embryos for those forms of breast, colon and ovarian cancer that run in families," predicts Arthur Caplan, Ph.D., director of the Center for Bioethics at the University of Pennsylvania in Philadelphia. Fears have been raised that the testing of genes might be just one short step from manipulating them—trying to make physical and personality characteristics that have nothing to do with disease prevention.

> *"In Italy a black woman and her Caucasian husband recently had a white baby using a donor egg."*

Caplan confirms that questions about shaping personality are likely to be raised in the wake of tests for such disorders as schizophrenia. He also foresees that in the next 20 years fertile couples might cruise the clinics "because we can forecast their babies' characteristics. If we don't put limits on who can offer these services, and on what sorts of traits people can pick, everything from 'Give me a tall blond child' to sex selection could be considered," says Caplan.

In Italy a black woman and her Caucasian husband recently had a white baby using a donor egg—to guarantee the child a life free of prejudice, they said. "This couple got their racial choice," says Caplan. "The question is: Should we be designing our descendants?"

What About Cloning?

In 1993 scientists at George Washington University in Washington, D.C., shattered a long-held ethical taboo by "cloning" a human embryo. That immediately raised the specter of human babies rolling off the assembly line—as well as of profiteering. "Down the pike, you could clone an embryo, put the genetic twin in the freezer and publish a catalog," muses George Annas, director of the law, medicine and ethics program at Boston University School of Medicine. "Anyone who wanted exactly that child could buy the embryo." Yet some doctors dismiss such possibilities. "It's not a technique that has any clinical usefulness based on the kind of work that's going on," says Dr. Wisot.

Embryo freezing, however, has already become fairly routine. Doctors store the "extras" produced during IVF so that couples can have another go-round at fertilization if the first attempt fails. Those embryos in the freezer are already creating daunting legal challenges.

"In Louisiana there's a statute that says an embryo in a petri dish is a person," notes Lori Andrews, who represented a couple in a suit against an IVF clinic that refused to return their embryo when they moved to another state. "They felt it was like dropping your kid off at day care and not getting it back," she says. "The court ruled they had the rights to the embryo."

Even more red flags are being raised about fetal issues. (An embryo becomes a fetus at the beginning of the ninth week of development.) In January 1994 Scottish researchers delivered baby mice from the eggs of aborted fetuses and announced that in a few years they expected to create human babies by this method. That raised the freakish possibility of women aborting their children and giving birth to their grandchildren instead.

It also ignited furious debate, with calls for a ban on the use of eggs from aborted fetuses in IVF. "Taking eggs from aborted human fetuses won't happen," says George Annas flatly. "It's too grotesque." Others disagree, envisioning "fetal farms," where women in need of cash can sell their aborted fetuses to black-market ova harvesters.

Although fetal farming may never become a reality, egg banking could. Dr. Howard W. Jones, co-founder of the Jones Institute for Reproductive Medicine in Norfolk, Virginia, discusses this possibility: "The egg is the largest cell in the body, and it doesn't freeze very well," he says, "but this problem could be solved in the next 5 or 10 years. If a woman wanted to postpone childbearing, she could have her eggs harvested and frozen, say, when she was 25."

Already, the issue of age-appropriate mothers is sparking heated debate. At Dr. Severino Antinori's fertility clinic in Rome, a 59-year-old British woman had a baby from donated eggs. . . . "There is concern about setting an age limit for women to have babies, particularly since France is already proposing limits," says attorney Lori Andrews.

What's needed, say Caplan and others on the front lines of reproductivity, is a wide-ranging public discussion of all these procreative options. As president of the American Association of Bioethics, Caplan will urge Congress to set up a national bioethics commission, comprised of doctors, lawyers and ordinary citizens. "When we're talking about a subject as basic as making babies," says Caplan, "everybody ought to be involved in the debate. We can still decide to make rules and shape how the technologies work. They haven't run amuck yet."

Reproductive Technologies Are Beneficial

by Jaroslav J. Marik

About the author: *Jaroslav J. Marik is a California physician who specializes in treating infertility.*

Family—religions, cultures, and traditions consider it to be the foundation of society, a unit necessary for the assurance of the continuous existence of humanity as we know it now and have known it in the past. Making this unit stronger and more stable is seen as the best way to secure progress and prosperity for the future.

The right of procreation is guaranteed by the Constitution, and Nature made sure that the process of procreation is closely connected to the loving relationship between a male and a female. The fruit of this love is what makes a family complete: a child.

From the beginning of our lives, we expect to become a part of this divine unit, when the right time arrives. Somehow it is automatically expected that we will become not only husbands and wives, but also parents.

It can be devastating to find out that parenthood may not be as simple and easy as we might have expected, and the thought that parenthood may never materialize might shatter our lives, our relations, and our future plans.

Lack of parenthood makes us feel unfairly denied the fulfillment of our existence. It gives us a feeling of personal inadequacy and failure stronger than any other failed dream or plan.

Thus completion of the family unit can change from the expression and exercise of love into very stressful days, months, and sometimes even years of our lives.

The medical profession has been aware of these situations for generations. Physicians know that a lack of parenthood can be as stressful as any other medical dysfunction, if not more so. I know very well; I have been treating infertile couples for more than twenty years.

Reprinted from Jaroslav J. Marik's Introduction to *Miracle Child: Genetic Mother, Surrogate Womb* by Cheryl Saban; ©1993 by Cheryl Saban; with permission of New Horizon Press.

Chapter 1

In early 1971, I met Dr. Ed Tyler and was introduced by him to this medical specialty. He had a special relationship with people who had difficulties with establishing a family. That was because he had experienced these difficulties himself, and he had done something about it—with multiple successes. "Doing something about it" should be the main moving power of couples with reproductive difficulties.

"Doing something about it" led to establishing sperm banking, various types of husband and donor inseminations, refined surgical techniques to correct anatomical changes in male and female reproductive systems, and the development of various medications for therapy of abnormal and improper functioning of these organs. Moreover, things have changed dramatically since the second half of the 1970s when Dr. Patrick Steptoe accomplished a pregnancy after the fertilization of a human egg outside of the female body. Unfortunately, the first such pregnancy ended in the uterine tube and had to be removed, but the possibility of human conception outside of the human body had been established. Shortly thereafter, successful conception was crowned by a live birth. Dr. Steptoe had recognized a problem and "done something about it." Since those days in the late 1970s, the understanding of human conception has progressed more than in many centuries prior to it and, with newly available options, has entered a new era.

Solving Problems

In the mid-1970s, a couple came to the Tyler Medical Clinic for a consultation about their situation and the available options to reach their goal—to have a child. After reviewing their case, there did not seem to be anything to offer; the wife simply could not become a mother. Then a question arose: Can some other woman, capable of motherhood, be inseminated with the husband's sperm, conceive and carry a child for them? My answer was prompt and definite: No. The second question followed: Why not? Now I did not have a prompt answer. After some more discussions and research, a team was formed, a suitable surrogate found, insemination performed, and a pregnancy, followed with a birth of a normal healthy child, accomplished. It was possibly the first such event in modern infertility medicine. The original couple had a problem and decided to "do something about it."

Since those days in the 1970s, more development in the field of modern reproductive technology has taken place. The established practice of sperm donation was enriched by the option of egg donation. Surrogacy was broadened by the employment of gestational surrogates to carry a pregnancy conceived by the sperm and the egg of the infertile couple. Furthermore, the fertilization of gametes assisted by various laboratory techniques became a specialty of its own.

The medical profession can now do much more than ever before and with much better success. If there is a problem, let's face it and "do something about it."

In Vitro Fertilization Benefits Infertile Couples

by Herbert A. Goldfarb, Zoe Graves, and Judith Greif

About the authors: *Herbert A. Goldfarb is an obstetrician/gynecologist and infertility specialist. He is a clinical instructor at New York University School of Medicine and director of the Montclair Reproductive Center. Zoe Graves is a medical writer. Judith Greif is a family nurse practitioner at Rutgers University Health Center in New Jersey and the author of the book* AIDS Care at Home.

> The difference between a successful person and others is not a lack of strength, not a lack of knowledge, but rather in a lack of will.
>
> *—Vincent T. Lombardi*

"I chose not to go to college because I figured it was a waste of time. I was going to marry the guy I was with in high school, so why bother spending my parents' money on college if I was going to have babies and stay home? It's not that I'm not a smart girl; I graduated with an academic diploma, but I couldn't see any use for a college education in my future."

Peggy never did marry her high school sweetheart, but later met Vinnie.

Peggy and Vinnie dated for two years before they got married. Although they used no contraceptives during this time, Peggy didn't conceive. She had had a similar experience with her high school boyfriend, whom she dated for eight years. "Nobody could be that lucky," she surmised. "Other girls, they go to bed, one-night stands, and suddenly there's a baby. Me, I could swing from chandeliers, and nothing."

The thought of being an unwed mother didn't bother Peggy. "I wouldn't have minded if I had a kid and nobody married me. 'You play, you pay and take the consequences' is my motto. I come from a good family. My parents weren't the type that would put me out on the street." Peggy was sure that there would always be a roof over her head. She started working at 14 years of age, and for seven years had a job as a teacher's aide in an elementary school. "I felt like I had my own set of kids over there," she recalls. The combination of a secure job and a supportive family made her feel safe and protected no matter what her future might hold.

After two years of dating, Vinnie and Peggy got married. It was another two years before the idea of having children came up. Even though Vinnie wasn't worried, Peggy knew she'd have a problem getting pregnant. "It's simple arithmetic," she told him, "Eight and four equals twelve plus zero. Eight years with my childhood sweetheart and four with you, is twelve plus zero kids." With that equation in mind, Peggy started seeing a gynecologist near her home. The process progressed very slowly. For six months, Peggy was instructed to monitor her temperature. She kept an accurate record of her basal body temperature, writing it on her chart every morning. When she saw her doctor, he told her that her charts looked okay, but he could not be sure if she was ovulating normally.

Searching for a Physician

Three months later, she was given a postcoital test to determine the quality and quantity of her cervical mucus and how well Vinnie's sperm could penetrate and swim through it. These tests were also fine. Another four months passed before the doctor decided to do an endometrial biopsy to examine the quality of the endometrial lining of the uterus.

"At that time, I used to live for home pregnancy tests," she said. "I ran on a relatively short cycle, so if I was so much as a minute late, I was sure I was pregnant. There were days when I would do two or three pregnancy tests a day. I used to hide them from my husband because they were 14 or 15 dollars each and I would spend 40 dollars a day easily on these tests."

The doctor informed Peggy that the endometrial biopsy was to be done on the 14th day of her cycle. However, after waiting a month for the day to come around, when she called the office, she was informed that the doctor was "all booked up." Frustrated and teary, she asked what would prevent the same thing from happening the next month. The receptionist curtly informed her that there was no guarantee that she would get an appointment then either. Peggy felt heartbroken and insisted on speaking directly to the doctor; she was sure he would be more understanding and flexible about fitting Peggy into her schedule. When she found the doctor to be even more abrupt and unyielding than the receptionist, Peggy requested she be given her records to use in her search for a new gynecologist.

"Ninety percent of infertility is correctable and 10 percent is unexplainable."

Peggy's dad was an electrical engineer for a nearby hospital. Since he'd been an employee at the hospital for over 20 years, Peggy thought he would be a great resource for finding a doctor who could give her the specialized help she needed. Her father did some research and gave her my name. At her first appointment, Peggy admonished me, "You can't go quickly enough. I hate for every cycle to go by, it just takes too long."

Because it had now been some time since her original gynecologist's tests, I felt some of them needed to be repeated and others added to the workup. Within six weeks, I had completed a battery of tests and examinations on Vinnie and Peggy that included blood tests, sperm studies, a new postcoital test and endometrial biopsy, and a hysterosalpingogram to check the state of the uterus and determine if the fallopian tubes were open.

No Obvious Cause of Infertility

Amazingly, all the test results were negative. Since the problem was not readily apparent, I recommended a laparoscopy. Peggy's colorful response to the recommendation was, "Lay me on the table, cut me open, do whatever you've got to do, just make sure I get a baby out of this." During the operation, I widened her fallopian tubes, which were slightly narrow, but much to Peggy's dismay, I was still unable to pinpoint the problem.

After the operation, Peggy was put on three cycles of clomiphene, one of the most common and effective fertility drugs. Then another hysterosalpingogram was performed to see if her tubes had remained open after the surgery. At that time, I discovered a small cyst, but still no noticeable cause of infertility was revealed.

One day after all of this, I announced to Peggy and Vinnie that I couldn't take their money anymore. "You're physically fine," I said,

> *"The odds were strongly against them."*

"Ninety percent of infertility is correctable and 10 percent is unexplainable. I have to put you in the unexplainable category. You could get pregnant tomorrow, you may not get pregnant for 10 years, or you may not get pregnant at all." But I couldn't let it go at that. I suggested that if they still actively wanted to pursue having a baby, they should try in vitro fertilization, a procedure in which a woman's eggs are fertilized outside her body and the fertilized embryos are returned to her uterus to mature. I directed them to an in vitro fertilization program that I knew was reputable and had good results.

At first, when Vinnie read the statistics and estimated the cost, he was indignant. "It's never going to work," he said. "We've got a 90 percent chance against us. It's like rolling down your car window and throwing $10,000 out. The odds are against us." But Peggy was adamant. "At least if we do this," she insisted, "we can say we tried everything."

The in vitro fertilization (IVF) program was so much in demand that the earliest appointment the couple could get was three months away. They were willing to wait. They were determined to give it a chance.

To prepare for the IVF, Peggy and Vinnie took care of all the necessary paperwork and educated themselves by attending classes and reading every pamphlet and article they found on the subject. The staff was willing to accept the testing I had conducted as accurate, so when the time for their appointment finally arrived, Peggy and Vinnie were more than ready to get started.

The doctor to whom I had referred Peggy and Vinnie was cautious about promising IVF success, warning that the odds were strongly against them. But Peggy and Vinnie already knew that, and wouldn't give up. To prepare her body for the in vitro fertilization, Peggy was given two daily injections, administered by her mother since Vinnie was too squeamish. The first, HmG, supplies hormones that initiate egg production and release. The other medication, leuprolide, works as a control for HmG in regulating the amount of hormones that circulate through the system. Each and every morning, Peggy drove quite a distance to the lab for an estrogen blood test to monitor the growth of her eggs. If she missed the 8 A.M. cutoff, it was too late, and she'd have to wait until the next day to have the test done, so she was up bright and early every day.

Getting Vinnie to supply the sperm was another problem Peggy had to deal with. He put up an objection each step of the way and she found herself trying to cajole him into giving a sperm sample. Sperm was needed for a semen analysis, and finally Peggy woke Vinnie up early one morning, got him into an aroused state, and then produced a bottle for him to deposit his sperm in. He was furious but his rage was allayed by the fact that when the results came back, they were above normal. "If 14 million was the normal count," Peggy announced, "his came back 42 million." Each time he had to produce a sperm sample, whether at home or at the lab, Vinnie put up a fuss. But he would ultimately give in. His strong, healthy sperm were an important element in the in vitro process.

Peggy was then scheduled for the first part of the procedure—aspiration of the ova. "The day they took out the eggs was traumatic for me. I was so upset that I was almost incoherent. They got seven good eggs but I had no idea if that was high or low. I thought that maybe seven was too few and they should have gotten twenty. 'Keep digging' I wanted to tell them, 'Go for twenty. I want a fighting chance.' In part of my mind I was sure it was not going to work no matter how many they took out. I was convinced it was a waste of time. The other part said, 'Keep trying.'

"It took two days to find out if the embryos developed—two very long days. I had to stop myself from calling the doctor 10 times a day to ask, 'What's going on over there with my incubating babies?' In the end, out of seven, one did not fertilize and one wasn't good because too many sperm had entered it. So that left five. They put

> *"In part of my mind I was sure it was not going to work. . . . The other part said, 'Keep trying.'"*

three of the embryos into my uterus and froze the other two as backup." Peggy was told that in this procedure, an average of six to eight eggs are usually retrieved, and three or four ready for fertilization was right in the ballpark.

Two days of bed rest was recommended following the insertion of the fertilized eggs in order to provide the best chance for implantation in the uterine wall. Peggy went a bit overboard, and decided not to leave the living room couch for the next two weeks, except to use the toilet. However, even after these extraordinary precautions, the results of the pregnancy test came back negative and Peggy felt devastated.

The Time to Be Brave

It took five months for Peggy to pull herself together enough to return to the program to have the second embryo transfer done. The process is referred to as a transfer when no eggs are being retrieved. By this time Peggy was feeling completely discouraged. She was comforted only by the fact that she had what she called "two possible babies." Peggy confided that she was afraid that once the embryos were reinserted they'd die and then she'd have nothing. That was why she had postponed the second in vitro fertilization attempt for so long. But the time had come to be brave, so she took what she felt was her final chance.

The day the doctor performed the second in vitro transfer, Peggy's youngest sister, who was seven years younger, gave birth to an eight-pound boy. Her mother was with the sister in Maryland and Vinnie had to be away for a few days on a business trip. Peggy felt completely alone. "I didn't begrudge my sister the baby, I just wanted my own and I felt abandoned by everybody."

Because Peggy had little hope for the success of the new implant, she relaxed only for the required few days this time and went back to work within the week. The night before she was due to return to the lab for the pregnancy test, she began bleeding. She was crying hysterically when she told Vinnie that the blood test for pregnancy was unnecessary—that she had her period and the second try had been a failure. The next morning she was going to go straight to work instead of stopping at the doctor's office for the test, but Vinnie objected. "If you don't get the test, the nurses are going to haunt you until you do," he said. "Even if you're right, they need to have the test results to prove that they're negative."

Despite the many years of gynecologists, infertility specialists, nurses and lab technicians, broken dreams and lasting disappointment, Peggy had remained calm, level-headed, and pleasant during her numerous visits. She had a reputation among the nurses for being exceptionally sensible and brave. "But that morning in the clinic after I had the pregnancy test, I lost it," Peggy said. "It's a good thing there were understanding doctors there or I think they would have called for a straitjacket for me. I began yelling, telling them I had enough. I screamed at everybody that I was bleeding, that I had my period and for them to get the charts out and do something for me, anything. I said I was not going through the same thing again with those needles and the waiting. The office full of doctors and nurses was silent as I stormed out of there."

Peggy drove straight to work, then left an hour later, too distraught to concentrate. That day, as she left work, someone sideswiped the new car Vinnie had given her the week before, and then sped away after informing her that he had no insurance. Peggy was so distracted that she never even got his license number. "I'm standing there, tears running down my face, thinking, 'I'm bleeding and there's no baby, I had an accident with a new car and nothing can go right for me.' I was like an animal. I rushed home so that I could compound the paint off the side of the car before Vinnie came home. I must have looked a wreck because my neighbor came over and gently asked what was the matter. I sobbed as I explained to him that I was trying to get the dent out of my car and that I wasn't having a baby."

> *"She was pregnant, although she had been the last to find out."*

Peggy went to see her sister, so she wouldn't have to be alone. At five o'clock, it was like an alarm went off in Peggy's head—time to get the results from the blood test. She couldn't bear to have them say she wasn't pregnant again so she put it off and wouldn't make the call. Finally, she asked her sister to make the call. Peggy was surprised as her sister asked the nurse, "Are you sure? Are you positive? You know she was bleeding, don't you?" Peggy dropped her glass as she reached for the phone. She could barely believe it as the nurse excitedly described how they had been trying to find her since the results came in at 2:30 that afternoon. Peggy was shocked as she heard the doctors call out their congratulations. The nurse told her that they had gotten the results early, and since they all knew how upset she was, they had been calling everyone they knew, to get in touch with her. By this time, her husband and mother had all heard the wonderful news. She was told that her husband had dropped the phone when he heard. She was pregnant, although she had been the last to find out. The doctor increased the progesterone medication she was taking because her blood level was a little low from the bleeding. Within four days, the bleeding had stopped.

But the worry had not ended. "Two days later they made me come in for another blood test. What for? Was I pregnant or not? Yes, but I needed a beta test which would tell if I might lose the baby. I couldn't believe it. The trouble didn't stop; being pregnant wasn't good enough. And now the beta test became just as important to me as the pregnancy test had been."

The beta-HCG is used to monitor the hormone level which is an indication that the embryo is still implanted in the uterus. The beta test results were fine. Then an ultrasound was performed to see how many embryos had taken. There had been two frozen embryos. Peggy said, "It didn't matter to me if they both took. Somebody took, that was what counted."

Like Winning the Lottery

But Peggy was not out of danger yet. For three months she had to go back every week for blood tests, ultrasounds, and other diagnostic tests. "You start off with a 90 percent chance that the in vitro is not going to work, and then once it works, three out of five women miscarry. How could I beat the odds? They were completely against me. When I hit the three-month mark, the end of the danger zone, it meant the baby was going to stick, and I was considered a normal pregnancy. Vinnie and I felt like we had won the lottery."

Other issues cropped up that didn't cause them to question their decision to have in vitro fertilization, but which did make it problematic. The first was that Peggy and Vinnie were practicing Catholics, and during the pregnancy, there was a controversy raging in the church concerning in vitro fertilization. They felt confused on the issue, but decided that the decision to go ahead was right for them.

Another worry Peggy had was that someone else's embryo might have mistakenly been used. "While I was having the transfer done," Peggy remembered, "the lady next to me was a woman named Elena Rodriquez. I thought, 'What if they mix the embryos up, if they put hers in me and mine in her?' I knew, no matter what, I wouldn't give the baby up! Even if it turned out that the baby had dark brown eyes while my husband and I have blue eyes, it would still be my baby."

"I didn't have much of a sense of humor about any of it," Peggy admitted. "Vinnie used to joke and say, since my embryos were frozen, if it was a boy, we should call him Chillie Willie, and if it was a girl, we would name her Crystal. I didn't find that funny but I didn't really care since my pregnancy was going so well.

> *"In the back of my mind was always the fear that something would go wrong."*

"But in the back of my mind was always the fear that something would go wrong—in vitro, frozen, chemicals— these were words that would shoot through my mind on a daily basis. I never truly felt out of danger."

For the rest of her pregnancy, Peggy transferred to a local doctor for her prenatal care. Peggy was petite and small-statured, weighing only 104 pounds before the pregnancy. Even though she gained over 60 pounds during the pregnancy, the doctor did not expect her to have a large baby, at least not over nine pounds, which was what her son turned out to be. After two days in labor, an emergency cesarean section was performed when it became clear that the baby was not coming out on its own.

Peggy and Vinnie could not believe what a perfect, healthy, and handsome son they had. And Peggy smiled to herself when the baby opened his eyes and she realized he had the bluest of blue eyes.

Miracles of Modern Science

Five months after Phillip was born, Peggy discovered she was pregnant again. No one could believe it! They had another boy whom they named James.

Chapter 1

Like his older brother, Jimmy had deep blue eyes, but while Phillip was blond, Jimmy had almost jet black hair. Jimmy was a quiet patient little guy, which made it easier for the couple to care for him and Phillip, who was not yet a year and a half old. The two boys quickly grew into strapping handsome toddlers, cheery and energetic.

Peggy and Vinnie still regard the birth of their sons not as merely good fortune, but as miracles of modern science. Nothing can compare with the amazement and gratitude that Vinnie and Peggy experienced on the birth of each of their sons.

The Catholic Church Should Support Reproductive Technologies

by Brian Doyle

About the author: *Brian Doyle is a writer and frequent contributor to* U.S. Catholic *magazine.*

I am lying on the floor watching my daughter, Lily, pick up a rattle. She is 3 months old and has never done this before. She regards the prey carefully for some minutes before suddenly sending her hands out on their expedition. The left hand arrives first; the right hand gets sidetracked and ends up caressing the carpet. After a brief period of uncertainty, her hand grips the rattle, and Lily hoists it into the air like a miniature barbell. She grins, a huge and toothless grin, and begins to chirp like a sparrow. I applaud; even the smallest miracles deserve recognition.

A baby, a rattle, and a fawning father are nothing new. All new parents are in-trinsically prone to musing about the miraculous, since new life is the most miraculous item on the menu. And although Lily's Herculean efforts to harness her motor skills are astonishing to me, they are only the opening notes of what will, I hope, be a continuous symphony of graceful acts. Why, then, do I feel that this first autonomous act is such an extraordinary little miracle? I feel this enormously. As I lie there on the floor, smiling and clapping gently, I can feel myself close to tears.

I think it is because I consider Lily herself to be a miracle of unusual propor-tions. She is a child conceived by *in vitro* fertilization (IVF), a "test-tube baby," in the harsh colloquial phrase of the day. She was not conceived in the warm womb of my tiny wife. She was conceived in a small glass dish in a suburban medical clinic a day after several eggs were taken from my wife's ovaries and several mil-lion sperm cells were contributed by me. From the dish she traveled by pipette back into my wife from whom she emerged mewling three months ago.

Brian Doyle, "The Church Shouldn't Prohibit Test-Tube Babies," *U.S. Catholic*, June 1992. Reprinted by permission of Claretian Publications, 205 W. Monroe St., Chicago, IL 60606.

Chapter 1

By the standards of the Roman Catholic Church, Lily is an unnatural child conceived by a "morally illicit" technique that separates procreation from the union of husband and wife. "The church remains opposed from the moral point of view to *in vitro* fertilization," concludes the "Instruction on Respect for Human Life in Its Origin and on the Dignity of Procreation," a publication issued by the Congregation for the Doctrine of the Faith in 1987.

The official opposition of the church to IVF rests on the guiding principle behind *Humanae vitae*, Pope Paul VI's 1968 encyclical; namely, that sex, love, and procreation are inseparable. Sexual intercourse is an expression of marital love, wrote Paul, and each sexual act must be generally open to the possibility of procreation. Because IVF divorces procreation from sexual union, it's wrong. In other words, a child conceived by means other than a loving sexual act is conceived illicitly from a moral standpoint.

There are other objections to the procedure. One is that the dignity of the new human life is violated by the intervention of the medical professionals who oversee fertilization and implant the embryo in the woman. Another is that the process sometimes entails the creation of several embryos, which are (depending on the IVF clinic) implanted all at once or frozen for later IVF efforts. To freeze an embryo is to treat life with disrespect, say church spokespersons; to allow several embryos to die *in utero* is what *New World* columnist Father John Dietzen calls "a deliberate destruction of human life."

> *"By the standards of the Roman Catholic Church, Lily is an unnatural child conceived by a 'morally illicit' technique."*

But it is on the inseparability of sex and procreation that the church rests its formal objection to IVF, says Father Richard McCormick, S.J. of the University of Notre Dame. "The church disapproves of IVF on the same grounds that it disapproves of contraception: that is, that love, sex, and procreation are inseparable. Because IVF separates sex and procreation, it's considered illicit, no matter what the circumstances may be."

Considering Cost and Morality

Let me tell you about the circumstances. My wife and I were married five years ago. Our marriage is rich and funny and poignant. We awaited children with trepidation and excitement, awed and thrilled at the chance to bathe a new soul in our coupled love. Month after month we hoped. Month after month we were disappointed. We went to a doctor to see whether there was a medical reason for our childlessness. There was; my wife's fallopian tubes were blocked by scar tissue. She had an operation to undo the damage; it only confirmed the permanence of the blockage.

I remember sitting in the doctor's office and hearing her say that we would not be able to have children of our own. I remember that her voice was gentle, but

34

that her words cut like razors. I remember that my wife's face grew sad and gray.

We registered with several adoption agencies; we got second and third and fourth opinions; my wife readied herself for more complicated surgical procedures; and we began to seriously consider *in vitro* fertilization. We thought about selfishness: at what point, we thought, are we pursuing parenthood too assiduously? When is it that you decide to stop trying to be the parents of your own child? We also thought about cost, about morality, and about the procedure's relatively low success rate (about 10 percent of women who undergo implantation of fertilized eggs give birth). And then we went ahead with the procedure.

> *"Lily . . . is holy beyond my comprehension and yours . . . and the pope's."*

A year later there is Lily.

"[IVF] is a subversion of the dignity and unity of marriage," says Dietzen in his column in the *New World*.

"[IVF] deprives human procreation of the dignity which is proper and connatural to it," say the authors of the "Instruction on Respect for Human Life in Its Origin and on the Dignity of Procreation."

"The child is not the fruit of intimacy, but the product of a scientific procedure," says Father John Connery, S.J. of Loyola University in Chicago, Illinois.

Lily makes another stab at the rattle again with her left hand. This time, however, she brings it slowly and carefully to her mouth. She spends the next few minutes happily trying to eat it.

Dignity, zygotes, subversion, illicit, procreation. Words, words, words. The reality is Lily, and she is holy beyond my comprehension and yours and Father Dietzen's and the authors of the "Instruction on Respect for Human Life in Its Origin and on the Dignity of Procreation," and the pope's. She is a miracle, pure and simple; and how she came about doesn't make a whole lot of difference to me. If holiness is in life—and that is the pervading principle of Christianity, the principle by which abortion is banned, the principle by which birth control is proscribed—then this life is holy, and to forbid the means by which it came about is, I think, foolish and cruel. Do we ban scientific intervention in other medical areas? Are heart transplants immoral? Are cesarean sections?

Drawing Lines

My anger at foolishness doesn't prevent me from understanding what well-meaning authors are trying to say when they staunchly defend the church's stance on IVF. We must adhere to principles, they say; otherwise, we're adrift in areas of incredible moral confusion. What about surrogate motherhood? What about donated sperm? What about genetic engineering? Where do we draw the line?

I don't know. But I sometimes think the church is very good at drawing lines.

Chapter 1

It seems to me that this particular line, the one drawn between married couples and their children, is a remarkably stupid one. It joins procreation and the conjugal act so tightly that it leaves no room for reality. My wife and I could not have children in the same way most parents have children. But now we have a child, a daughter so gentle and beautiful she breaks my heart every day. Did we do something wrong? The church tells me that the procedure by which Lily came to be is morally illicit. I disagree; I think it is a miracle, and I think the church hierarchy is lost in a dusty corner of the Moral Mansion, far away from where people live and far away from the things people carry in their hearts.

Having thoroughly gummed her rattle, Lily is now absorbed in the clowns tattooed on her blanket. She waves her fingers over them like a tiny magician. I chirp, just for fun, and Lily looks up at me. We stare at each other for a moment. On her face an enormous smile appears. She laughs, a sound like the crisp note of an alto saxophone, and my heart breaks again into thousands of pieces.

I laugh, too, and then I begin to clap gently. I do so because I think miracles should be applauded, not forbidden.

Reproductive Technologies Harm Women

by Robyn Rowland

About the author: *Robyn Rowland is a social psychologist and senior lecturer in women's studies at Deakin University in Geelong, Victoria, Australia. She has contributed to the books* Test-Tube Women: What Future for Motherhood? *and* Man-Made Women: How Reproductive Technology Affects Women. *She is the author of the book* Living Laboratories: Women and Reproductive Technologies, *from which this viewpoint is excerpted.*

Imagine women coming to maturity in the next century—less than a decade away. According to Gena Corea:

> These will be women who, from their earliest days, grew up with IVF, embryo transfer, surrogate motherhood, artificial wombs, and sex predetermination technologies. They will be women who have never known a world without 'superovulation' and 'ovum capture'. From childhood, these women will have watched television news reports involving the 'Storage Authority', that is, the board in charge of frozen sperm, eggs and human embryos.

> They will be women whose own 'mothers' may have supplied the egg from which they were generated, *or* the uterus in which they were gestated, or perhaps neither. These women of 2050 will know that among women, there are egg donors and there are breeders or gestators and there are those who provide various body parts and fluids used in reproduction (for example, urine from which hormones are extracted for use in superovulating the ovaries of younger females). But no one woman procreates a baby all by herself. This will be so because by 2050, use of the new reproductive technologies will have expanded beyond the original category of women—the infertile—for whom it was first touted.

> This, then, might be the reproductive consciousness of our daughters in the 21st century: 'Reproduction is a complicated intellectual and technical feat performed by teams of highly skilled men who use, as raw material for their achievements, the body parts of a variety of interchangeable females'.

This vision of our future may seem shocking, yet it is certainly feasible. When talking to high-school students about reproductive technology I usually end by looking at a conversation a journalist had with Dr Brinsmead of Newcastle University in which he said: 'A fetus that is not even born could ultimately have children'. He explained that immature eggs could be harvested from a female fetus at its fourteenth week, brought to maturity, mixed with sperm, and used to create a child. At the moment, students respond to this with disgust, calling it 'repulsive', 'horrifying' and 'unnatural'. They are shocked and revolted, just as their

> *"Step by step, we are . . . eroding the control which women have had over procreation."*

parents would have been merely ten years ago if they knew that by the 1990s there would be storage banks of frozen human embryos in most major countries of the world. Yet the same students readily accept the existence of these banks and the fact that sexual intercourse is not the only way of having children. Already their sense of how humans are created is vastly different from that of their parents—just as ours is different from our parents'. We have all been affected by the softening-up processes which mould our reproductive consciousness, reshaping our sense of how people are and should be created. Few people in the 1990s blink when they hear the words 'test-tube babies', and terms like 'in vitro fertilisation' (IVF) and 'cloning' are commonly used even though it is less than two decades since the first IVF baby was born in England.

Yet despite the continuing development of the new reproductive technologies, people remain basically in the dark about how they work and about the continuing research which pushes so-called benign technologies into the more bizarre areas like Brinsmead's concept of the 'fetal mother'. They are not aware of the high failure rates and costs of the technologies both to individuals and society. The social effects are masked because the technologies are presented as a solution to individual problems. Subtly, step by step, we are changing the nature of being human and eroding the control which women have had over procreation. In its place, male-controlled technological intervention is beginning to determine how children will be conceived, what kind of children will be born, and who is worthy of receiving these new products of our science.

Commodification and Control

There is a common belief that ideas or theories are somehow separate entities inhabiting a place called academia, remote from reality. So the scientific control of reproductive technology is often debated as if it is an intellectual exercise, while in the laboratory and in the market place increasing scientific control over procreation continues. At the same time we accept an increasing commodification of all things. Education, knowledge, information are now 'products' to be bought and sold, along with the new 'products of conception'—which used to be called 'children'. Even the 'self' is packaged and marketed in courses on how to 'sell yourself'. The ideology of family is used to sell reproductive technology, with babies up front as the sales pitch. Babies sell products; babies become products. One newspaper account exemplifies this when discussing so-called 'surrogate' mothers:

> Its first product is due for delivery today. Twelve others are on the way and an additional 20 have been ordered. The 'company' is Surrogate Mothering Ltd and the 'product' is babies.

The precedent for this has been the packaging and selling of woman as object. Advertising uses women's bodies and sexual availability this way, and an entire industry of pornography reaps its profit from this objectification. With the new reproductive technologies women are further objectified and fragmented, dismembered into ovaries and eggs for exchange and wombs for rent. The commodity 'woman' or a part of woman can be used to produce the commodity 'child'. And the product had better be perfect. As Herbert Krimmel wrote, 'It is human nature, that when one pays money, one expects value'.

The product will be 'man-made' (*sic*) and therefore better than nature; and because our society does not accept the imperfect, women will be placed under more and more pressure to use all technological means offered to secure perfection. Less and less assistance will go to those who make the 'mistake' of having an imperfect child. So in the age of the perfect product, difference (named 'defect' or 'abnormality') will be less and less acceptable.

Implicit in this is our increasing desire for control—control over nature, genetic problems, difference, ageing, death and fertility. Men in power, the makers of ideas and systems of control, construct a make-believe world in which 'free choice' exists, in which individuals supposedly make choices about their lives unhindered by social responsibility to others. In this view of society, the way power works is subtly hidden behind claims for personal autonomy.

The Myth of Control

Belief in human control is used in order to reduce human fear of risk. But risk—risk of being hurt, of death, of a handicapped child, of a sudden disability or illness—is in the nature of life. The 'control myth', the myth that we have choice, leads people to believe that they are free, that there is no need to challenge those in power. It also places responsibility for the downside of the world—poverty, illness, domestic violence—on the individual and not on structures of power. The illusion of freedom is a powerful control mechanism.

> *"Male-controlled technological intervention is beginning to determine how children will be conceived."*

Though our whole society is changed by the new reproductive technologies, initially they affect women most intimately. A history can be traced of the continuing battle between the two social groups, men and women, over the control of women's fertility and procreative potential. This battle is also drawn around race and class lines, and governments constantly develop systems structured to control which women have children, when, how and how many. The new reproductive technologies extend their power to do so in ways unimaginable a few decades ago. . . .

Men and the Control of Reproduction

Historically, there has been increasing control by men over women's reproduction. There is a history of the elimination of women healers by a rising male-dominated medical profession and the encroaching of this profession into women's control of birth. That control, extending to control over pregnancy and now conception itself, has dangerous implications for women. . . .

Womb Envy

In an analysis of consciousness, the male desire for control springs from male alienation from childbirth and procreation. Psychoanalysts have written extensively on the theme of womb envy. Freud's case studies document fantasies by men and boys for women's organs and functions. Anecdotal data abound concerning boys' desires to develop breasts and to give birth. Men's fascination with and envy of women's procreative ability has also been represented in myth and rituals. For example, in some societies *couvade* is the male imitation of childbirth which can include the mutilation of the penis to resemble a vagina and male imitation of the pain of childbirth to the point where the father-to-be actually takes to his bed. Myth also represents male desire to control reproduction. The Greek god Zeus gave birth to the goddess Athena by swallowing her mother and giving birth to her through his head; he also sewed Dionysus into his thigh in order to carry that pregnancy to term.

"With the new reproductive technologies women are further objectified and fragmented."

Though men initially thought the mystery of pregnancy and birth lay entirely within women's hands, once they realised they had a role by delivering the seed, they attempted to inflate this role. Early scientific anatomists actually concealed their observations that women contributed to the fetus. 'Their rationale was that as Nature had hidden from sight the sexual organs of women, so women's contribution to a new life also should be concealed.' In the seventeenth and eighteenth centuries, scientists developed the belief that sperm carried within it the minuscule human being, the homunculus. The woman was merely a vessel that cared for the developing male seed.

Men and women experience reproductive consciousness differently. The fact that men provide only the seed in reproduction ensures what Mary O'Brien calls their alienation from genetic continuity. Because women bear the child and labour at birth, they have had (until recently anyway) the certainty of their essential participation. As Carole Pateman has written:

> No uncertainty can exist about knowledge of maternity. A woman who gives birth is a mother, and a woman cannot help but know that she has given birth; maternity is a natural and a social fact. . . . Unlike maternity, paternity is merely a social fact, a human invention.

Men, excluded from this certainty, have tried to annul their alienation from reproduction by the 'appropriation of the child'. O'Brien sees this experience reflected in obstetrics to which men have brought 'the sense of their own alienated parental experience of reproduction, and have translated this into the forms and languages of an "objective science".'

This alienation can generate a frustration which results in 'feelings of inadequacy, jealousy or hostility toward the female'; women are immortal in a way in which men are not. Women can regenerate themselves, but men need women in order to regenerate themselves. Azizah al-Hibri argues that men remake 'the female's womb and breasts, making them his and divorcing them from their biological functions' in sexual appropriation.

Men Increasingly Control Pregnancy

These theories of alienation and envy in reproductive consciousness resulting in male control and violence towards women can be explored in the elimination of midwives by male midwives in the nineteenth century. That development represented the beginning of male-dominated medical control over pregnancy and birth. Through modern reproductive technology men limit their alienation and increase their control further. They are now capable of conception itself. They can take the egg in their hands and inject the sperm into the egg through micro-injection techniques. In this sense they become symbolically both mother and father to the in-vitro-created child. A man can rent a woman's womb to carry his child for him and in what Carole Pateman describes as 'a spectacular twist of the patriarchal screw, the surrogacy contract enables a man to present his wife with the ultimate gift—a child'.

Importantly, as men decrease their alienation by appropriating conception itself—taking women's eggs from their bodies—they alienate women from their own reproductive processes, changing the certainty women once had about reproduction. No woman on a reproductive technology programme can know for sure that the egg or embryo placed back inside her body was that which came from her body.

"Our whole society is changed by the new reproductive technologies."

Men are also appropriating the self of woman through this process. This is most obvious in the slavery of so-called 'surrogate' motherhood. The man is not buying merely a service, but the woman herself. The service cannot be delivered unless the woman herself is delivered. According to Pateman:

> The self of the 'surrogate' mother is at stake in a more profound sense still. The 'surrogate' mother contracts out rights over the unique physiological, emotional and creative capacity of her body, that is to say of herself as a woman.

Finally, the male desire for control of reproduction lies also in the nature of power itself. Being the dominant group, men expect to control all social resources, including reproduction. But women, the subordinate group, have had exclusive control over the process of pregnancy and birth. Men may deliver the seed but it is the processes of a woman's body which bring the embryo to fetal life, and then produce a live child. Men have only been able to experience that vicariously through women's discussions of it. Men cannot accept their exclusion and have constructed institutions to invade that realm of women's experience.

"Anecdotal data abound concerning boys' desires to develop breasts and to give birth."

The Power of Procreation

Supported by the ideology of the 'patriarchal family', the 'control myths' of self-sacrificing motherhood and womanhood, and male definitions of women as irrational, incompetent, defective, dangerous and an object to the male subject, men as a social group are using the vehicles of science, medicine and commerce to establish control over procreation. It is therefore within the power dynamic of the oppressed and the oppressor that men will not allow women to retain their monopoly over reproduction and birth. Discussing 'surrogacy', Pateman writes that

> men have denied significance to women's unique bodily capacity, have appropriated it and transmuted it into masculine political genesis. . . . Thanks to the power of the creative political medium of contract, men can appropriate physical genesis too. . . . Now motherhood has been separated from womanhood— and the separation expands patriarchal right. Here is another variant of the contradiction of slavery. A woman can be a 'surrogate' mother, only because her womanhood is deemed irrelevant and she is declared an 'individual' performing a service.

Procreation and birth are a resource which women have and men want. All forms of creativity carry a certain power; in this instance, the resource of another human being is created as well as the subject of love and affection. Like all groups who 'own' a capacity such as this, women want to hold onto their exclusivity, which is part of the group identity of women. They are the group that has the potential for giving life. In a world in which not a great deal belongs to women, this has been something which does. If what was offered to women was a sharing in the joy and creativity and limited power of procreation and birth, they might view men's desire to enter the reproductive arena differently. But as it expresses itself in a destructive and woman-hating invasion of women and their bodies, it can never be welcomed.

In the process of trying to end their own alienation, men have made procreative alienation a reality for women, divorcing women from their wombs, eggs and embryos—from their own bodily selves and their sense of procreative continuity. They have made children products of the nexus between commerce, science and medicine, calling experimentation on women and human society 'therapy' and camouflaging the intention to map and control human genetics with the rhetoric of 'helping the infertile'. In this process women have become the experimental raw material in the masculine desire to control the creation of life; patriarchy's living laboratories.

Reproductive Technologies Are Open to Abuse

by Ellen Goodman

About the author: *Ellen Goodman is an author and nationally syndicated columnist.*

How do you describe the theft of a human egg? The kidnapping of an embryo? The abduction of reproduction?

Start by imagining, if you will, that you are an infertile couple who wanted a biological child badly enough to go through the expense, the indignities, the emotional and hormonal roller coaster of in vitro fertilization. Imagine the month-by-month hopes and disappointments.

Imagine discovering years later that you do have a child. A boy born to another couple from your egg and possibly your sperm. Or twins carrying your DNA but someone else's name.

Imagine discovering that the "extra" eggs harvested from your body and maybe fertilized by your sperm were cavalierly given to another pair without your knowledge, without your permission. Your genetic material had been "donated" to them by your doctor.

This is the bizarre tale unfolding in California, where two couples are accusing doctors of theft and fraud. But these alleged burglaries didn't take place at some fly-by-night medical office, or by some unknown quack.

This scandal of staggering proportions is said to have occurred at a renowned fertility center at UC Irvine. The doctor being charged is Ricardo Asch, the very man who devised the GIFT [gamete intrafallopian transfer] procedure that greatly increased the odds of success of in vitro fertilization—the man who also helped one of the suing couples give birth.

Asch, along with two partners, is accused of many things, of using unapproved fertility drugs and failing to report thousands of dollars to the university. But the charge that strikes the deepest is that he used eggs and sperm, fresh and frozen embryos, as if they were his to distribute.

Ellen Goodman, "An Ethical Time Bomb Explodes," *San Diego Union-Tribune*, January 10, 1995; ©1995, The Boston Globe Newspaper Company/Washington Post Writers Group. Reprinted with permission.

Asch denies all this. He claims to be the victim of extortionists. But along with the mounting evidence accumulating in seven different investigations against him, there is a sense of a story that was waiting to happen.

In 1980 the first act of creation took place in a laboratory. The reproductive possibilities that followed the birth of Baby Louise have made our heads spin.

In these years, reproductive "material" has been separated from what we used to think of as the reproductive process. We've seen an egg and a sperm that got together in a petri dish implanted in a third person's womb. We've seen surrogate wombs, postmenopausal mothers, women giving birth to their own grandchildren.

One result has been the joy of 40,000 couples who became parents. Another has been the dashed hopes of many more who didn't beat the long odds against success. But an unsettling byproduct of laboratory creation has been the extra embryos, the spare eggs and sperm, the DNA frozen in suspended animation, ready or not for some later use.

In the past decade, a couple who died in a plane crash left their embryo in a freezer and left their relatives in a quandary. Another couple sued each other for custody of a frozen embryo as the last remains of their dissolving marriage.

We are also warehousing all sorts of genetic material—who knows how many embryos, how many eggs, how many vials of sperm?—from infertility treatments. In a desire to alleviate the desperation and pain of childlessness, we have walked waist-deep into an ethical quagmire.

How hard would it be for a doctor trained to think about eggs as "reproductive material" to decide not to "waste" the leftover "material"? How hard would it be for a doctor whose single goal was to make babies to make them any way he could? This is a field, after all, with remarkably little oversight and even less regulation. Wasn't it likely to happen?

Too Little Caution

I am not suggesting that egg- or embryo-napping is somehow understandable. This is not in the ethical gray area. If the charges are true, Asch broke every rule in the book, from the guidelines of informed consent to the laws against burglary. If so, he violated the trust of his patients, violated their bodies and family bonds. If so, he's a thief, plain and simple.

But even if this is a rogue doctor, the fact is that infertility treatment is a medical business typified by too much desperation and far too little caution. It's wide open to abuse.

Today, that's become as clear as a crystal petri dish. One of the stars of the field is now charged with the cruelest and most perverse of ironies. He's accused of tricking infertile couples, who wanted nothing more than to have their own children, into providing children for others. And there are at least four people left wondering about what one anguished father calls "the missing children."

Sperm Donation Undermines the Family

by John Leo

About the author: *John Leo is a contributing editor of* U.S. News & World Report *and a nationally syndicated columnist.*

David Blankenhorn has a question: Why isn't there some debate about the fact that American sperm banks sell sperm to single women?

As usual, the elite culture in America will hear this question in one way; the rest of the country will hear it differently.

Elite response: Here comes another attack on privacy and individual rights, particularly the right of women to control their own bodies. Besides, it insults women to imply that they need a man around to raise a healthy child.

Rest of the country: Why is it so obvious that a wide-open commercial market in the production of fatherless children is a social good? The consensus of studies is that no-father children, as a group, are at risk in all races and at all income levels. If so, doesn't society have a stake in discouraging the intentional creation of fatherless children, in suburbs as much as in the inner city?

A Casual Attitude

Mr. Blankenhorn is head of the Institute for American Values in Manhattan. While researching his new book, *Fatherless America*, he fielded many queries from journalists about the practice of selling sperm to single women. He said virtually every question came from Japanese or European reporters who were shocked that the United States is so casual about a free market in sperm.

Other nations have indeed taken the issue more seriously. France banned the sale of sperm to single women. Britain allows it. Japan makes it difficult, but not impossible, for single women to acquire donor sperm. Italy has no law, but in April 1995 its national association of doctors voted to deny artificial insemination to single women. European guidelines, produced by the Council of Europe in 1989, say sperm should be made available only to heterosexual couples.

Why has serious moral debate occurred in other developed nations, but not here, where most of the world's sperm banks are located? Well, for one thing, the United States is the only nation that discusses almost all its social issues in "rights talk," a language with a built-in tendency to grant individuals un-trumpable rights against even the most sensible social policy. The American "rights" dialect is so pervasive that even its opponents are usually required to speak it (in this case by arguing that children have a "right" to have a fa-ther around.)

> *"Fathers and fatherhood have virtually dropped out of the literature and the discussion of reproductive matters."*

The abortion wars played a part too. The sharp focus on women's rights and choice was inevitable, but part of the psychic fallout has been a tendency to downplay the role of the male, as if the father had no stake at all in the fate of the fetus or reproductive issues in general. Feminists, some strongly hostile, have been prone to portray all procreative issues as principally a female concern. Fathers and fatherhood have virtually dropped out of the literature and the discussion of reproductive matters. In an age of antagonism between the sexes, it's a short step here to the view of fathers as troublesome, marginal and essentially irrelevant inseminators.

Alas, the American open market in sperm, virtually unquestioned and undis-cussed, institutionalizes this view of the irrelevant male. Men can spawn chil-dren with no responsibility. Women can raise them without putting up with a male. Writing in the *Utah Law Review*, Daniel Callahan, bioethicist and head of the Hastings Center, sees "an acceptance of the systematic downgrading of fa-therhood brought about by the introduction of anonymous sperm donors. [It is] symbolic of the devaluation of fatherhood."

A Threat to the Family

People on the other side of this non-debate understand what's at stake. Here is John Edwards, a sociologist at VPI, writing in the *Journal of Marriage and the Family:* Sperm donation "purposely makes paternity problematic. . . . In theory, the new reproductive technologies signal the obsolescence of marriage and the family . . . implicitly the innovations suggest that the family of the future may merely consist of one socialized adult and an offspring."

Biological fatherhood was once understood by society to carry with it perma-nent moral obligations to the child. Now it can involve nothing more than a fi-nancially strapped college student masturbating into a cup for $50 and writing a vaguely caring letter to an offspring he will never see or care about.

Messrs. Edwards and Callahan are basically saying the same thing: Artificial insemination of single women is not just about ticking biological clocks and the urgent desire to have a child; it is, in fact, an expression of a whole new social policy that turns away from the ideal of an intact family toward what we used to call a non-intact or broken one.

This is the most glaring example of what Daniel Patrick Moynihan calls "defining deviancy down." Take a devastating social problem—fatherlessness—and redefine it as an acceptable and even inevitable model for the future. In this new model, the father is either infantilized, absent or simply dropped out of decision-making and nurturance. In any of these cases, male irresponsibility is basically licensed and legitimated. Before this model gets more firmly established, let's have a real national debate.

Infertile Couples Should Pursue Adoption, Not Reproductive Technologies

by Sallie Tisdale

About the author: *Sallie Tisdale is a contributing editor for* Harper's Magazine *and the author of* Talk Dirty to Me: An Intimate Philosphy of Sex.

The urge for children can be terribly fierce and, thwarted, terribly hard. My reproductive equipment went awry when I was still a teenager. Young, unmarried, I got pregnant in spite of all the conflicting medical advice I'd received. I gave birth a month before my twenty-first birthday and had a hysterectomy before my twenty-second. I struggled through years of grief over my hysterectomy, grief mixed with changing degrees of anger and self-pity. I mourned the children I would never have, the lost womb. In the effort to avoid a hysterectomy, I'd had a D&C, a hysterosalpingogram and several laparoscopies, and if I'd had more procedures to choose from, I might have tried more. My hunger for another child was deep; it was also simplistic. "Child" required "pregnancy." Eight years later, married, I adopted two children from Guatemala, a toddler girl and a boy of nine. And now I can't imagine subjecting myself, or encouraging any woman I know to subject herself, to the pain and risks and costs of infertility treatment. We will believe that parenthood through pregnancy is somehow better—somehow more *parental*—until it is proven otherwise to us. My adopted children have given me this proof.

Letting Go of a Dream

Adoption is often dismissed by people in infertility treatment as difficult or expensive or risky. It's no more so than infertility treatments, often less so. Neither comes with guarantees; both require repeated self-examination. I found adoption to be such a deliberate process that it was frightening. I had so many chances to turn back. I had to work for that unseen, wanted child. In contrast, a

Sallie Tisdale, "Biological Motherhood—Is It Better?" Reprinted, with permission, from the May 1993 issue of *Glamour*.

pregnancy seems almost casual.

After my surgery, adoption seemed unreal, a distant, almost meaningless prospect. I simply fretted—if only I could have another child. If only. Turning to adoption means letting go of a dream, letting go of the child we have imagined who will be like us, of us. And that turning takes time.

Finally I met a woman who had had eight miscarriages before adopting. She asked me, "Do you want to be pregnant, or do you want to have a child?" When I thought back, I saw that the pregnancy and labor, though hardly benign events, hadn't changed me. But the child that resulted changed me and my life's path forever. So did the second child. So did the third.

Opening Your Heart

Some people believe they won't be able to feel love for a child who looks different, who comes from "somewhere else." But the dream of the imagined child dies with every birth. After pregnancy, a person comes into your life, and many first-time mothers comment on how surprised they are at that new person's personality—its individuality. The newborn is, unexpectedly, a stranger. In adoption there comes a point similar to birth, a moment when a real child is presented—through a photograph, a description, or simply whole and alive. To accept that child as your own and become its *parent* means opening a new place in the heart. You are, either way, forced out of yourself into the world. Suddenly all children seem more alike than different. Suddenly all the children of the world are your children.

The Right to Reproduce

Every decision we make about reproduction in a crowded and hungry world is a moral decision. I know many people defend their obsession with infertility treatment as a right: the right to reproduce. But I wonder if they understand what that must mean. Infertility is at least as common among the poor as it is among those wealthy enough to afford medical help. Does this "right" really extend only to the tiny, largely white and relatively affluent population that can afford high-tech medical intervention? And what are the rights of the children already here, whom no one wanted in the first place?

> *"I can't imagine subjecting myself . . . to the pain and risks and costs of infertility treatment."*

I didn't know that millions of children in this world live in conditions of extreme poverty, hunger and pain until I started looking for a child to adopt. I *knew*, but I didn't really know, until I saw where my children came from, heard the stories of other adopted children and children still without families. Now I flinch when I hear or read of a "shortage of babies" for adoption in this country. What a reprehensible phrase. In the United States many pregnant women don't get basic prenatal care, and many children grow up unwanted, endangered and malnourished. In much of the rest of the world babies die by the thousands for lack of a few cents' worth of protein. I no longer believe people have a right to reproduce themselves; instead, I think all people have the right to be parents. The right I believe in, and want to champion, is the right of children already among us to have good nutrition, education, shelter—and families.

Chapter 2

Should Postmenopausal Women Become Pregnant?

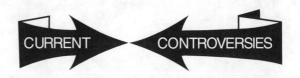

Pregnancy and Postmenopausal Women: An Overview

by Sandi Dolbee

About the author: *Sandi Dolbee is the religion and ethics editor of* The San Diego Union-Tribune *newspaper.*

In the book of Genesis, Sarah, eavesdropping on a conversation between the Lord and her husband, Abraham, hears that she is going to have a baby.

She laughs.

According to the Old Testament story, Sarah is 90, long past her childbearing days, and Abraham is 100. But within the year, she gives birth to Isaac.

Now, centuries later, science has replaced the biblical miracles of fertility, and society finds itself swept up in an ethical debate over how old is too old to be a mother.

"Is it right to intentionally create children if you know that both parents are likely to be entering a nursing home before the kid is in elementary school?" asks Arthur Caplan, director of the center for biomedical ethics at the University of Minnesota.

"I think it would be an imprudent and immoral public policy to intentionally create orphans."

But others argue that it is not that simple.

Like the bitter debate over abortion, the complicated questions sparked by the 59-year-old British woman giving birth to twins in December 1993 through artificial conception is steeped in the conflict between individual choice, concerns for the child and fears of what unbridled science might bring next.

Now, a 61-year-old Italian woman, helped by the same doctor, is pregnant.

"This calls for the principle of equal consideration," says John Quiring, assistant director of the Center for Process Studies, a theological think tank at Claremont School of Theology.

Sandi Dolbee, "Debates for the Ages—Motherhood After Menopause: A Testament to Science or Selfishness?" *San Diego Union-Tribune*, January 11, 1994. Reprinted with permission from the *San Diego Union-Tribune*.

"Consideration of the quality of life for the infant, the mother, the father, the society. It's just not the issue of the two people who want to bring another life into the world—or the one person."

A key question for Quiring, along with other ethicists and behaviorists, is whether the parents are going to be around to take care of the child.

"Since the life expectancy is 72 for men and 78 for women, can they support a child through adolescence?" Quiring asks. "The risk that they won't is fairly high."

> *"A key question . . . is whether the parents are going to be around to take care of the child."*

"None of us has a contract with God," counters Ashley Phillips, executive director of Womancare, a San Diego women's health clinic. "I am a mother and could be hit by a truck tomorrow. That's why I have life insurance.

"As a feminist health-care provider, I believe it is the woman's choice to get pregnant and I support it. At the same time, I'm concerned that it takes incredible medical resources to make it happen in a world where many people are not getting the medical care they need."

Regarding the risk that the child will end up motherless or dependent on society, "We like to give women a little more credit than that," says Jennifer Coburn, San Diego spokeswoman for the National Organization for Women.

"They are the most appropriate people to weigh the possibilities and make the choice."

Issue of Selfishness

But some behaviorists argue that people have become too narcissistic, their choices are selfish ones, based too much on self-gratification and too little on the needs of others or the long-term effects.

"It seems to me that it is necessary to consider that children should not be had for the sake of a mother," says Dr. Melvin Goldzband, a San Diego psychiatrist who sits on the bioethics committees for Sharp HealthCare and the San Diego County Medical Society.

"Children should be had for the sake of children."

That is too often a novel concept in today's society—regardless of the parent's age, Goldzband admits.

"Having a child is not the same as having a Ferrari or having a beautiful home or having a face lift," he says. "Having a child is making a commitment to someone else."

Goldzband argues that each woman should be evaluated physically and emotionally before being accepted as a candidate for artificial fertilization.

"I would suspect that most women, not all women, . . . who decide to have children at advanced ages have reasons for doing this that are inside themselves. The welfare of the child is not as important to these women underneath as their own gratification is."

He is among those who also worry what these children will become, growing up in a home in which the parents are two generations removed.

"I think we are going to have a society of children reared by exhausted parents . . . who simply lack the wherewithal to keep up with their children, to care for their children and to continue giving to their children in a way that younger parents can," he said.

But Cecil Steppe, director of the county Health and Human Services Department, is not so sure.

Steppe cautions not to generalize beyond the data—and the data in his welfare office show that grandparents who have stepped in to raise their children's children are doing a pretty good job.

Besides, says Steppe, who will turn 61, he thinks he probably would be a better father now than he was when he and his five children were younger.

"I think our system is backwards to begin with," Steppe suggests. "We have our children when we are least emotionally and financially capable typically."

The Double Standard

There is, of course, a double standard in this issue, notes Italian fertility specialist Dr. Severino Antinori, who impregnated both women in Europe using the eggs of younger women fertilized by the sperm from the women's husbands.

"A man can have a child at that age and everyone says, 'Isn't he clever.' But those same people say a woman of 55 is a dishrag," Antinori told reporters.

But Caplan, the Minnesota ethicist, says: "I can't help it if older men find younger women and have babies with them. That may not be wise, but at least there is a shot that a child has one parent.

"If older men and older women together have children, it's not the same thing."

Conservative, traditional religions—from Roman Catholicism to Orthodox Judaism—agree with Caplan. The issue for them is not so much age but what they regard as ungodly biological manipulation.

"The fact is, it is not her egg, it is not her child," says Rabbi Moishe Leider of Chabad of La Jolla.

Still, ethicists are reluctant to make this issue a matter of public policy.

"Having a child is not the same as having a Ferrari or having a beautiful home or having a face lift."

"I think this is a matter that should be carefully weighed by people who are involved as individuals," says Clifford Gorbstein, professor emeritus of biological science and public policy at UCSD. "I would not have a law to set some kind of limit."

David Anast, publisher of the *Biomedical Market Newsletter* based in Costa Mesa, says:

While I appreciate and share some of the current concerns regarding this issue, I feel that ultimately the government has no legal or moral right to interject itself into the decision-making process of when and if to have children, when and if to get married or other personal, family matters.

Agreeing is the county's Steppe: "We need to voice our opinions, but then it is an individual issue. Just like abortion, it would be an individual issue."

Dr. Antinori has said he will not accept a woman unless she has a life expectancy of 19 more years. Mark Sauer, a fertility doctor at USC, has an informal age cap of 55.

As for Sarah, the elderly mother portrayed in Genesis, the Bible says she lived for 37 years after having Isaac, dying at the age of 127. Abraham, the father, died a few years later.

Having Babies After Menopause Would Benefit Women

by Margaret Carlson

About the author: *Margaret Carlson is a Washington, D.C., correspondent for the weekly newsmagazine* Time.

On Christmas Day 1993, a 59-year-old British woman gave birth, making her the world's oldest known mother of twins. Two days later in Italy, an even older woman, Rossana Dalla Corte, 63, announced that she too would give birth to a baby in June. Both women had pursued their pregnancies for the most tender of reasons. Dalla Corte and her 65-year-old husband lost their only child, then 18, in a motorcycle accident three years ago. Jennifer F., as the British press dubbed her, a successful businesswoman and a millionaire, decided belatedly that she had missed the fulfillment of having a child. By slipping the physical coils of menopause, these women have inspired not just wonder but an intense debate over the question of when a woman is too old to become a mother.

Britain gave its answer in the case of Jennifer F., denying her fertility treatments on the basis of age. She went to Italy, where gynecologist Dr. Severino Antinori says he has helped 47 women over the age of 50 give birth at his Rome clinic. In the U.S. most doctors and clinics have already answered the question by parceling out the limited space in in-vitro fertilization programs to women under 45 on the grounds that younger women are more likely to succeed in the program and would be less prone to complications.

Indeed, the health risks of being pregnant at 50 are greater than those at 30, but careful monitoring minimizes those risks. Older mothers using donated eggs give birth to babies that do just as well as those born to younger women, according to Dr. Mark Sauer, a fertility expert at the University of Southern California.

Those who oppose such treatment appear to have reasons other than medical for denying motherhood to older women. When doctors in London refused to treat Jennifer F., they told her that they believed she was too old to face the stress of being a mother. In defending the decision, the British Secretary of Health said, "There are deep ethical considerations, and the child's welfare must be considered. A child has a right to a suitable home."

Dr. Arthur Caplan of the University of Minnesota argues that children have a right to a mother who won't be heading to a nursing home just as they are heading for high school. But what about men on Metamucil and pacemakers who become fathers? Senator Strom Thurmond, who had four children in his 60s and 70s, and Charlie Chaplin, who was 73 when he fathered his last child, did not have to seek approval when they sired their offspring. By the thousands, men over 45 exercise their perpetual rights to fatherhood, marrying and remarrying, having first and second families, without challenge to their right to do so. When it is a man having the baby, few seem to question whether the stress will be too much for the old geezer. One could contend that the assertion that a child is worse off with a mother who may die before the child is grown than a father who might is an argument for more equal parenting.

> *"Older mothers using donated eggs give birth to babies that do just as well as those born to younger women."*

Those who cheer for Jennifer F. point out that society is not always kind to women as they age. A young woman might be discriminated against; an older woman is often seen as irrelevant. Actresses have complained for years that their male counterparts don't run into the same career roadblocks they do once they reach 40, but the dilemma is more serious than whether Meryl Streep is in as much demand as Jack Nicholson. Lauren Hutton and stories about older women and younger men notwithstanding, the woman who can no longer give birth may sometimes feel as used up in modern America as she was in preindustrial times, when bearing children was a key to economic survival.

The capacity to bear a child is one of the most powerful forces shaping male-female relationships. Certainly the biggest difference between men and women in their late 30s is that women see a deadline for procreating creeping up and men don't. This difference affects the way women approach work—their peak childbearing years usually coincide with their make-or-break career years—as well as the dating game. Instead of looking at men casually, with that insouciance so valued by the Letterman generation, panicky women for whom the biological clock is tolling evaluate each prospect for his potential as a father. This one-sided pressure to mate alters the social firmament. The very act of needing to be married and to have a child before it is too late may keep a woman from reaching her goal; a woman for whom time is running out may send out the wrong signals.

One argument against older women having children is that both parents will be too old to do the job right or to see their kids grow up. But that presumes that older women will always marry men their age or older. Once it is more acceptable for women over 45 to have children, the pool of men open to them expands. Then younger men who want to start families may feel freer to fall in love with older women. For those couples, there indeed could be better living through chemistry.

Older Mothers Can Be Excellent Parents

by Linda Wolfe

About the author: *Linda Wolfe is a writer and author of the book* Double Life.

In 1990, my brother, then 62, announced he was going to have a baby.

His wife, in her 30s, was childless. She had long wanted a child, but my brother, who had a 26-year-old son, feared he was too old.

Now, he had decided to go for it.

What I remember most clearly from our conversation was jealousy—not the sibling rivalry that had dogged his days and mine but something larger. A railing-at-the-gods kind: Why should he still be able to make babies when I, half a decade younger and much more of a nurturer, was doomed to post-menopausal shutdown?

So it was with a delight bordering on the passionate that I heard about the 59-year-old British woman who gave birth to twins by virtue of eggs fertilized by her younger husband and implanted by Italian doctors.

And it was with an indignation bordering on the painful that I learned she was the object of ethical debate centering on whether a woman that old ought to be a parent.

A Double Standard

Who debated the ethics of my brother's having a baby—little Alex, now nearly 4—who will finish eighth grade when his father is 75 and graduate from college when his father is 83?

I heard little debate when, in the early 1980s, the spectacular rates of divorce and remarriage began to make it common for men with children in their 20s to start new families.

When these men sired their new children, their reproductive feat was celebrated, not criticized—and then emulated.

Now, medical technology enables women—just a few, all apparently super-healthy and super-rich—to have babies late in life. Suddenly, there's a hue and cry.

Older mothers! They'll be in nursing homes before the kids are out of school! They'll be dead! Even if they live until their children reach adulthood, their off-spring will be psychologically damaged.

If a child is going to have an older parent, an older mother is a better bet than an older father. The statistics say she's going to live seven years longer than he.

Will she be in a nursing home while her child is small? Highly unlikely. The average age of women seeking babies through the new technology is 51. The average age of people entering nursing homes is nearly 85.

Older and Better

There is no evidence in the psychological literature to indicate that older parents are unfit parents. In fact, some evidence suggests that because they tend to bring economic tranquility and emotional stability to baby-rearing, they are better parents.

Such advantages, not to mention the blissful enthusiasm for parenthood that is the hallmark of most graying mothers and fathers, may outweigh drawbacks associated with anxiety about health and stamina.

Women of a certain age always have helped rear America's children. How many children are being reared by grandmothers? Hundreds of thousands? Millions? Are the grandmothers too old for the job? Should we take the children from them? Of course not.

> *"If a child is going to have an older parent, an older mother is a better bet than an older father."*

Some critics maintain that when older people have babies, they disrupt the proper order of things—that there is a time to procreate and a time to give it up.

OK, but only if all those potential daddies in their 50s and 60s are willing to give up the privilege, too. And you can bet they never will.

To criticize older women, who are having their shot at it, while admiring or accepting the profusion of older daddies is blatant sexism.

Just because science makes something possible doesn't mean it's unethical. Think of the heart surgery that has helped millions of people, many of them older daddies, live beyond the time that nature might have granted them.

Pregnancy After Menopause Can Be Medically Safe

by Mark V. Sauer, Richard J. Paulson, and Rogerio A. Lobo

About the authors: *Mark V. Sauer, Richard J. Paulson, and Rogerio A. Lobo are physicians who specialize in treating infertility.*

Women of advanced reproductive age may become pregnant after in-vitro fertilisation of oocytes donated by younger women, followed by transfer of embryos. Previous reports have focused on pregnancies in menopausal and perimenopausal patients less than 50 years of age, but women over 50 years also request our help to become pregnant. That practitioners are reluctant to establish pregnancies in older women is evidenced by the observation that very few centres in the USA provide such a service (< 5%). Indeed, until recently, women over the age of 40 were also not generally accepted for oocyte donation. Nonetheless, our data indicated that these women retained uterine receptivity to embryo implantation. . . .

Since in older women the uterus responds adequately to steroid hormone replacement therapy, the only barrier to pregnancy seems to be the physical and psychological health of potential recipients. Thus, we devised criteria for and extended our protocol to an even older group of recipients. Here, we report our preliminary experience of embryo donation to women beyond the age of 50 years.

Results

The protocol for oocyte donation and embryo transfer to women over 50 years of age (mean [SD] 52.2 years [2.5]; range 50–59) was approved by the Institutional Review Board of the California Medical Center, Los Angeles. . . .

Between April, 1991, and August, 1992, there were . . . 21 embryo transfers to 14 recipients.

Excerpted from "Pregnancy After Age 50" by Mark V. Sauer, Richard J. Paulson, and Rogerio A. Lobo, *Lancet* 341 (February 6, 1993):321–23; ©1993 by The Lancet. Reprinted with permission.

Pregnancies were established in 9 women, 1 of whom had a preclinical loss. In another woman an anembryonic [no embryo] pregnancy was diagnosed at 7 weeks' gestation; medications were discontinued and the pregnancy self terminated.

A low overall fertilisation rate was noted. On the basis of abnormal semen analyses with 0% hamster egg penetration, we considered that there was a "male factor" in 5 couples before the in-vitro fertilisation attempt; in 1, no fertilisation occurred. Although a single pregnancy was established by 1 of the 5 couples, most (98/152; 64%) of the non-fertilised eggs occurred in this subgroup.

The obstetric outcome of the women delivered is as follows:

Total clinical pregnancies	8
Spontaneous abortions	1 (anembryonic 7 week spontaneous abortion)
Deliveries	3
Continuing pregnancies	4
Gestational age at delivery	37 weeks; induced vaginal delivery
	35 weeks; caesarean section; preeclampsia, twin gestation
	35 weeks; growth retardation; preeclampsia
Multiple gestations (twins)	2
Caeserean section births	2 of 3 delivered
Obstetric complications (*)	
Preterm labour	1
Preeclampsia	2
Growth retardation	1
Gestational diabetes	1

(*) Total of 5 events in 2 patients.

To date there have been no serious complications. Of the 7 pregnant or delivered women, 4 had never previously conceived. The remaining 2 are grandmothers.

Discussion

This study clearly shows that women well beyond natural menopause may still achieve adequate uterine receptivity to allow implantation of transferred embryos. Our trial of embryo transfer to this population was founded upon the observation that the uterus can be maintained in a receptive state for embryo implantation well beyond the ovaries' ability to provide normal gametes to reproduce or the hormonal sustenance to support an early pregnancy.

> *"Establishing pregnancy in individuals nearing 60 years of age becomes a . . . rational goal."*

Observation has caused us and others to conclude previously that the ageing ovaries, not the uterus, are responsible for most adverse fertility events at least up to the age of 49 years. Thus, we pos-

63

tulated that the enhanced pregnancy wastage rates seen in spontaneously conceiving women over 40 years is due not to an adverse uterine environment, but to abnormal embryogenesis [formation of the embryo]. This conclusion is supported by the high incidence of aneuploidy [abnormal number of chromosomes] seen in offspring and abortuses of women in this age range.

To fully assess differences that might occur in implantation rates, we decided to transfer our usual number of embryos (4–5) back to these older patients. Although the risk for multiple gestation increases with this practice in younger patients, there is no other way to fully evaluate an age effect on implantation unless a standardised approach to embryo transfer within the programme was maintained. In the rodent, ageing and normal implantation and early embryonic development are inversely related. However, the rodent model may not be applicable to man or other primates. No data for women beyond 50 years of age are available since spontaneous pregnancy in this age group is a rare natural event. Since normal . . . responses are observed in the endometria of older women prepared for oocyte donation, we feel it is likely that early pregnancy events will progress normally in this group of individuals.

Although there have been no serious complications, there are not enough data at this time to presume that the incidence of adverse results will not increase. Since prevalence of most obstetric complications increases in women even in their late 30s, one would expect an even greater risk in our older group. Careful precycle

> *"It is unlikely that this new technology will have a serious influence on the fabric of the society."*

medical screening may prevent the inadvertent inclusion of patients with known diseases, especially those with cardiovascular and diabetic complications. Intense monitoring during pregnancy may also lessen the probability that a disorder will go unrecognised. To reduce the chance of late adverse events, such as preeclampsia, abruptico placentae, or stillbirth, we recommend timely delivery after the fetus reaches maturity (about 37–38 weeks' gestation).

A Rational Goal

The psychological effect of giving birth beyond age 50 is unknown. Although little is known about the effect of age on parenting, the couples enrolled in this study appeared emotionally and physically well-equipped to meet the challenge. Certainly, many children have been raised by grandparents in various cultures. Prospective analysis of these families will be required to fully assess the impact of bringing a newborn baby into the lives of couples of advanced age.

As the average life expectancy and quality of life in our population increases, establishing pregnancy in individuals nearing 60 years of age becomes a more rational goal. In the past, only men have had the option of becoming parents in their 50s and beyond. Physiology kept this opportunity away from women.

Since few individuals choose to become parents late in life, we believe that it is unlikely that this new technology will have a serious influence on the fabric of the society, other than to open new doors and possibilities to some people.

There is little doubt that the uterus remains receptive to embryo implantation and development of normal pregnancy well beyond the limits of natural reproduction. This observation strongly suggests that the great majority of pregnancy wastage experienced in women in their fourth and fifth decades is due to the adverse effects of age on the oocyte. Our study casts further doubts on the existence of a "uterine factor" in infertility, at least with respect to the natural biology of ageing through the sixth decade. Women who wish to become pregnant in their 50s should be rigorously screened medically and psychologically, and if found to be fit, the option of oocyte donation should not be withheld.

Postmenopausal Women Should Not Become Pregnant

by Ana Veciana-Suarez

About the author: *Ana Veciana-Suarez is a reporter for the Knight-Ridder/ Tribune News Service.*

Some parents pray for wisdom, others for happiness. A few implore for money. I, I pray for strength and stamina.

That is why I have been following, with equal parts curiosity and disbelief, news reports about post-menopausal women who have spent small fortunes trying to get pregnant.

Do they know what they're getting into?

Technology now permits a normally infertile woman to be implanted with another woman's fertilized egg, and a small but growing number who can afford the many thousands of dollars it requires are choosing to do so. A 62-year-old Italian is expecting. A 59-year-old British woman gave birth to twins in December 1993, and so did a 51-year-old Israeli, six years past menopause.

I am convinced they do not know—cannot imagine—the endurance needed to raise a child.

I am convinced they have not looked 10, 15 years hence.

I am convinced that they are thinking of themselves and not their children.

Or, as French Health Minister Philippe Douste-Blazy so aptly put it: "For me it is totally shocking to see a child whose mother will be 80 when he is 18. This seems to me totally undeserved. I think that when you undertake a pregnancy you cannot be egotistical; you have to think first of the child."

Wreaking Havoc

Science can work wonders. It can produce test-tube babies, surrogate mothers, cloning and genetic engineering. It can give hope—and wreak havoc. Unfortu-

Ana Veciana-Suarez, "Ability to Give Birth After Menopause Doesn't Make It Right," Knight-Ridder News Service, January 18, 1994. Reprinted by permission: Tribune Media Services.

nately, unwittingly, we may be creating more of the latter without appropriate measures to control and curb this nascent field of reproductive technology.

There's a lot more to parenthood than pregnancy and childbirth, much more than 2 a.m. feedings and running around the playground. A 50-year-old woman considering bearing and raising a child must look beyond the fuzzy and warm vignette of an infant in a receiving blanket, beyond the bassinet days and pre-school and homework and ballet classes. Parenting involves caring and guiding and loving and being there past infancy, through the chaos of adolescence and into the triumph of adulthood.

> *"It is totally shocking to see a child whose mother will be 80 when he is 18."*

Imagine being 65 with a 15-year-old. Imagine paying for braces and college on Social Security.

Not a pretty picture. Not a logical, natural one, either.

It happens sometimes, of course, nature pushing the boundaries. On these very rare occasions, women in their late 40s have mistaken pregnancy for the onset of menopause. But deliberately getting pregnant at such a late age is a different matter. We do not have a God-given right to reproduce, but we do have a responsibility to be there for our children, to meet their needs when they are 12 as well as when they are 2.

Some fertility specialists claim that regulating insemination procedures is tinged with sexism. They cite the example of older men who have become fathers well beyond their prime. "When Charlie Chaplin has a child at 70, we say it's wonderful," complained a French fertility specialist. "But when a woman—who has a higher life expectancy than a man—has a child at 52 . . . that strikes us as terrible."

Because men have been doing it doesn't make it right. I would say the very same thing to them: Stop thinking about yourself. Consider the child.

Nature Is Wise

Nature knew what it was doing when it set its own cutoff date for childbearing. It wasn't trying to be arbitrary, just logical.

Natural evolution protects us from ourselves, whether or not we understand or like it. An older woman's body cannot handle the strains of pregnancy as well as when she was younger, nor can she handle the long, arduous labor of raising a child—and long and arduous and labor is exactly what child-rearing is all about.

There is, I know, the deep and abiding pain of infertility, the very real need of some women to nurture and care for a child—reasons often cited for pursuing, at incredible monetary, moral and emotional costs, a much-wanted pregnancy. But there are also many, many children in need of parents, children eager and willing and ready for adoption. We need to think of them, too.

Chapter 2

"Society encourages an obsession about the biological child," laments Elizabeth Bartholet, Harvard law professor and author of *Family Bonds: Adoption and the Politics of Parenting*.

Biological mother of one and adoptive mother to two, she points out that these babies born of implanted eggs are not genetically related to the mother. In fact, they are the newest form of adoption. Is it then fair to bring another baby into the world for the sake of experiencing pregnancy and birth, for our own shortsighted, selfish pleasure, when there are so many children waiting?

No.

Just because we can doesn't mean we should.

Society Will Be Harmed If Postmenopausal Women Are Allowed to Become Pregnant

by John Leo

About the author: *John Leo is a columnist for* U.S. News & World Report, *a weekly newsmagazine.*

"Never do everything that's possible" was the slogan of Howard Gossage, an advertising man prominent in the 1960s. That saying comes to mind as the smiling face of Rosanna Della Corte beams forth from newspapers and television. She is about to become the oldest woman ever to give birth. At age 62, she is pregnant, courtesy of advanced medical technology.

In London, a 59-year-old woman gave birth to twins as a result of the same technique: Multiple embryos, formed from borrowed eggs and a partner's sperm, are implanted in the hope that at least one embryo will survive.

Mrs. Della Corte, who wants to replace a 19-year-old son who died in an auto accident, will take her place in the Guinness Book of World Records. But records are meant to be broken, as the sportswriters say, so inevitably even older women will follow as high-tech mothers.

What's wrong with this? Well, in addition to the familiar problems of surrogacy (these women are basically overaged surrogate mothers who intend to keep their children), there is the obvious moral problem of manufacturing children they won't be around to rear and protect. By the time the kids are ready for kindergarten, Mom and Dad may be ready for a nursing home.

Actuarial tables being what they are, the children are likely to be parentless before puberty. If women try this technique at ever higher ages, the medical personnel involved will, in effect, be in the business of creating orphans. The fact that the technique often results in multiple births will just add to the victim count.

Dr. Sandy MacAra, chairman of the Council of the British Medical Association, thinks having post-menopausal babies at a quite advanced age is just fine, because "relative youth is no guarantee of parental function or competence. . . . Better, it may be argued, a fit, healthy 59-year-old than an unfit, unhealthy 19-year-old."

Alas, this is feel-good rhetoric. Rearing children is an exhausting long-term responsibility, and no sane society should encourage people to start undertaking it on the brink of old age. MacAra would have been better off saying plainly that medical technology now allows self-indulgent consumerism among baby-minded oldsters.

"Rights" Talk

So far, much of the defense of high-age motherhood has been conducted in "rights talk" (people have the right to do whatever they wish with their own reproductive systems). Rights talk is a familiar impediment to moral discussion. In this case, even opponents of high-age birth use the language: "Women do not have the right to have a child; the child has a right to a suitable home," said the British secretary of health, Virginia Bottomley.

> *"By the time the kids are ready for kindergarten, Mom and Dad may be ready for a nursing home."*

But rights talk almost inevitably leads to the cordoning off of a social issue as somehow private and beyond moral discussion. Anyone who converts a wish or a claim into a "right" usually wins whatever game is being played by inventing a trump card.

Those who see this issue as a morally troubling one have to start by throwing out the newly minted trump: There is no unassailable "right" to use high-tech reproduction techniques at age 60, 70 or 80, any more than there is a "right to a suitable home." It's a social issue as well as a private one, because society has to speak for the children involved.

Some women have raised the issue of sexual equality: Men in their 60s commonly become new fathers. Why is it wrong for women and right for men?

Short answer: It isn't, or shouldn't be. For men, becoming a father at an advanced age is largely a byproduct of a second marriage to a younger woman. This has won wide social acceptance, but the problem is the same as for Rosanna Della Corte: One parent, at least, is likely to die before the crucial work of parenting is done.

There are obvious echoes here of the spreading debate over single-parent homes. Either you believe parenting is a two-person job or you don't. If you do—and the evidence supports this view—then the same principles have to be applied to Rosanna Della Corte as to teenaged girls in the inner city. If parents can't plausibly promise to stick around 17 or 20 years until the job is done, they just shouldn't procreate.

A Better Use of Money and Resources

The social view, rather than the "rights" view, is all the more important when society is asked to foot the bill for high-tech birth experiments. It makes no sense at all for the public to fund expensive adventures in overaged baby-making when health costs are breaking the bank.

Society may not be able to stop the rich from indulging themselves, but it certainly can withhold public funds and try to shame doctors into making better use of their time and talent.

Right now, there's little likelihood of risky reproductive experiments being covered in national health plans, but never underestimate the mix of compassion and rights talk. The "right" to get something, and to get it paid for, can materialize very quickly around dubious but highly publicized desires.

Chapter 3

Is Surrogate Motherhood Beneficial or Harmful?

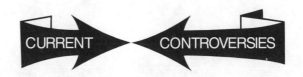

Surrogate Motherhood: An Overview

by Margot C.J. Mabie

About the author: *Margot C.J. Mabie has written several nonfiction books for young adults and articles for an adult audience. She is a teacher and editor and the author of the book* Bioethics and the New Medical Technology, *from which this viewpoint is excerpted.*

Of all the new forms of procreation, perhaps the best known and most discussed is surrogate motherhood. In surrogacy a woman carries a child for another couple, to whom she turns the child over upon birth.

In 1984 Mary Beth Whitehead read an ad for women interested in surrogacy. The mother of two children, she had enjoyed her pregnancies and thought that surrogacy offered her a good way to help a couple who could not bear children. And so she applied to, and was accepted by, the program run by Noel Keane, a lawyer who had come to specialize in the business of matching surrogates with couples who were unable to have children. Whitehead signed a contract by which she agreed to be inseminated with William Stern's semen and carry the child to birth. Because there were no laws pertaining to surrogacy, adoption laws would be used; Whitehead would terminate her parental rights, and Elizabeth Stern would then adopt the child.

Keane's services did not come cheap. His share was $10,000. Whitehead would receive $10,000 upon the delivery of a live, healthy baby. But in the case of Whitehead and the Sterns, the financial costs were trifling compared with the emotional costs. Their deal went awry when Whitehead fell in love with her baby. She and her husband fled with their two children and the baby girl in a desperate attempt to keep the infant. They were found by the police in Florida, and the baby was taken back to New Jersey, where the Sterns took custody of her. The Whiteheads went home to New Jersey and began the long legal battle to regain the child.

The mystique of motherhood, along with the biological fact that it is the mother, not the father, who carries and bears a child, was for many a justification of Whitehead's stronger claim to the child. Here the term *surrogacy* was a misnomer. Whitehead was no stand-in. She was the child's genetic, as well as gestational, mother.

To weaken that claim, others pointed out that Whitehead had signed a contract to act as a surrogate for the Sterns. A deal is a deal, they insisted. Further, the Sterns could offer Baby M, as the baby was referred to in the course of the legal proceedings, a

> *"The very idea of surrogacy was foreign and unsettling."*

better life. The Whiteheads' marriage was shaky—indeed, during the legal battle the Whiteheads separated and later divorced. Richard Whitehead had had problems with alcoholism, and neither had any higher education. Richard Whitehead was a garbage collector, and Mary Beth Whitehead had at one time been a go-go dancer. In contrast, the Sterns were professionals, she a pediatrician and he a biochemist. Their marriage appeared strong and calm. The Sterns could give the child a richer environment—richer intellectually and monetarily. The argument over who would be better parents was carried to the absurd when a psychologist, Marshall Schecter, testifying as an expert witness, said that Whitehead was not a good mother because she had not played pattycake properly. Instead of clapping at the end of the rhyme, she had said, "Hooray!"

Harvey Sorkow, the lower court judge who first heard the case, ruled that Whitehead's contract with the Sterns was valid and enforceable. He terminated Whitehead's parental rights and immediately carried out adoption proceedings by which Elizabeth Stern became the child's mother. The case was immediately appealed to the New Jersey Supreme Court, which ruled that Whitehead's parental rights could not be terminated against her will, and while custody of Baby M remained with the Sterns, Whitehead was given visitation rights.

Challenging Old Assumptions

The case, closely covered by a swarm of reporters from media across the country, was arresting. Many people had been unaware that surrogacy even existed, and while the medical technology—artificial insemination—by which this surrogacy was effected is neither high-tech nor new, the very idea of surrogacy was foreign and unsettling. What was new was the open, high-finance deal making surrounding surrogacy, a crass challenge to age-old assumptions about what makes a family a family. Hilary Hanafan, a psychologist who works with surrogate mothers, plumbs the public's bemusement:

> I think surrogate parenting . . . really is a direct threat to each individual's notion about their own relationship with their mother. . . . Surrogate parenting is a very threatening concept in the sense that it questions whether or not a mother's attachment to her child is absolute.

That class was so manifestly a part of the arguments about who would be better parents for Baby M gave credence to the charges made by opponents of surrogacy. They see surrogacy as nothing more than baby selling. They hold that the fees paid to surrogates are simply a means of exploiting women who need money, and they envision a society in which the rich pay the poor to serve as baby factories. When all is said and done, the $10,000 a surrogate might earn for bearing a child is a pittance.

Feminists, looking at surrogacy not so much as rich versus poor but as men versus women, are divided about surrogacy. Many assert that it is yet another way to demean women by placing them in a mechanistic role. They worry that surrogacy will come to be used by couples in which the wife views pregnancy as inconvenient, scary, risky. Indeed, Elizabeth Stern was not infertile. She chose surrogacy on the assumption that a self-diagnosed case of multiple sclerosis might be exacerbated by a pregnancy.

That surrogacy can spell misery for all the participants is amply demonstrated by the Baby M case, but there are many women who have been surrogates and have found the process rewarding. "It's a gift to be able to give others the same joy of a child that my husband and I have in our son," one surrogate said. They reject the view that surrogacy should be banned, pointing out that prohibiting it demeans women because any restrictions are (paternalistically) predicated on the idea that women are not intelligent enough to decide how they will run their own lives, make their own happiness. And they reject the notion that this is nothing more than baby selling, a desperate gambit for women financially up against the wall. The fees paid to surrogates are perfectly appropriate recompense for their work. "The money is not the most important thing," one surrogate explained, "but it has let me stay home and be a full-time mother, which is very rewarding."

Gestational Surrogates

In another form of surrogacy the surrogate is only the gestational mother. If a woman has ovaries but no uterus, she and her husband can use IVF to create an embryo, which is then implanted in the uterus of a woman who is willing to carry the child to birth. That was what Mark and Crispina Calvert did, but Anna Johnson, their surrogate, eventually balked, just as Mary Beth Whitehead had. In the ensuing custody suit, a California judge ruled in favor of the Calverts. Further, Johnson was not given visitation rights. Is Johnson's case truly weaker because, as the judge pointed out, unlike Whitehead, she was not also the genetic mother?

> *"There are many women who have been surrogates and have found the process rewarding."*

Suppose a couple wanting a child arrange for the creation of an embryo from donated egg and donated sperm, to be placed in the uterus of yet another woman for gestation. Whose claim to be the mother is the strongest? How shall we rank all these forms of motherhood?

By any reckoning, the procreative technologies have led to a mind-boggling array of possible mother-child relationships. A child can have three mothers: a genetic mother, the woman who provided the ovum; a gestational mother, the woman who nurtured the child in her womb before birth; and a social mother, the woman who raises the child.

Who is the child's true mother? Feminist Barbara Katz Rothman believes pregnancy is the key:

> Any pregnant woman is the mother of the child she bears. Her gestational relationship establishes motherhood. We will not accept the idea that we can look at a woman, heavy with child, and say the child is not hers. The fetus is part of the woman's body, regardless of the source of the egg and sperm.

By Rothman's standard, Mary Beth Whitehead and Anna Johnson were ill-treated by the judicial system; they are the true mothers of the children they bore. . . .

Babies or Products?

The overarching issues that arise from surrogacy and AID [artificial insemination with donated sperm] concern the meaning of a child and the meaning of the family. Critics of surrogacy point out that the fee paid to the surrogate is not for services but for a healthy baby. Whitehead's contract provided for payment of only $1,000 if the baby was stillborn. Further, the contract gave the Sterns the right to demand that Whitehead have an abortion if prenatal testing indicated that the fetus was in any way less than perfect. What are the children of these arrangements? Are they the expression of our reverence for and delight in life, or are they mere goods in a commercial transaction?

> *"The procreative technologies have led to a mind-boggling array of possible mother-child relationships."*

Many people believe that surrogacy and AID allow parenthood to slip from its essential mooring in the family. They worry that a subtle dynamic can come into play between parents who do not have a parallel relationship to their child. If the adorable baby has an obstreperous adolescence, will one parent find it easy to wash his or her hands of the problem, charging, "This child isn't mine"? And what of the covenant of marriage, by which people bind themselves together in a relationship of emotional and sexual constancy? Ethicist Paul Ramsey believes that that covenant is violated by procreative techniques that provide a husband and wife with only an illusion of true genetic parenthood:

> Most Protestants, and nowadays a great many Catholics, endorse contraceptive devices which separate the sex *act* as an act of love from whatever tendency there may be in the act . . . toward the engendering of a child. But they do *not* separate the sphere or realm of their personal love from the sphere or realm of their procreation, nor do they distinguish between *the person* with whom the

bond of love is nourished and *the person* with whom procreation may be brought into exercise.

Ethicist Joseph Fletcher disagrees. Constancy in marriage, Fletcher asserts, is not necessarily defined by constancy in procreation. It is love, not genes, that gives parenthood its meaning and richness. His defense of AID holds as well for surrogacy: "Insemination from a donor is not adultery if marriage fidelity is conceived . . . to be a personal rather than a merely legal relationship."

The technology that can change the way we conceive, carry, and bear children is itself in its infancy. . . . How we respond to the ethical questions that the currently available and the potential technologies pose will describe our views about the purpose and worth of marriage and the family, as well as the purpose and worth of the individual.

Surrogate Motherhood Is Beneficial

by Cheryl Saban

About the author: *Cheryl Saban is a writer who lives in California. She and her husband, Haim, have a son and a daughter from surrogate mothers.*

When my two precious miracle children are old enough to understand, I will tell them the story about their incredible births. I will recount the feelings of love and determination that inspired us to search for a way to have them. I will let them know that their very existence was made possible by a dedicated group effort, specifically by the unselfish, benevolent actions of two of the most charitable women I know. Kathy and Lori will always be a part of my life.

But just as their participation in the birth of my children was vital, their gentle retreat to the sidelines has allowed my husband and me to get on with the job of parenting. They happily accept the relationship of "fairy godmothers" in the lives of our children and do not feel left out in any way, as all of our lives resume normalcy.

Nevertheless, these spectacular moments in time have been etched in stone. None of us will ever forget them, nor will we ever be the same. This kind of love touches you deep in the core of your soul, and the warm glow of happy remembrance is never far below the surface. As each day passes, I look upon the smiling faces of my children, and I am continually overwhelmed by the magic of it all.

A Half-Full Glass

In retrospect, it's impossible to know what I would have done, or how I may have reacted, had we not been able to achieve our goals so quickly. I sadly realize that this is the case at least 80 percent of the time.

There is a voice inside of me, however, that says that had I not been successful so swiftly, I would have stubbornly continued the drug therapy, the surgeries, the mood swings, the surrogate search, the anxiety, the drama, the waiting, and the hoping to try to achieve that elusive pregnancy with a surrogate.

And, it seems, I would find myself in good company. Most infertile couples who seek an alternative to parenthood against all odds *think* they will succeed. They tend to see the glass as half-full, as opposed to half-empty.

In our case, I know that the end justified the means, and our positive attitude proved to be prophetic. The triumphant end result has brought us so much joy that the nearly uncharted road we traveled to attempt this controversial alternative to parenthood was more than worth the effort. In fact, I would call it priceless.

Procreation, this most primitive of instincts, exists in us all and is triggered in thousands of hopeful couples every day. However, there are just as many couples who cannot consummate their dreams, no matter how strongly they yearn.

The desire to parent a child sends approximately 3.5 million couples each year on the quest of their lives. For them, one of the most innocent and natural acts of our human existence is denied. Many times they don't know who to turn to, nor do they know how far they should go with their search. It can be one of the most frustrating, emotionally challenging, and marriage-threatening experiences a couple can go through.

Thankfully, this search leads many couples to adoption, which is still a wonderful option, for both the child and the adoptive couple. Children who are raised by adoptive parents can delight in the fact that they were wanted so desperately, and loved so much, that a special search was made to find them.

Whether one seeks to adopt a child in the traditional sense, utilize artificial insemination, or achieve parenthood through surrogacy and IVF, the legacy of love is as strong and cherished as it could possibly be.

I'm not trying to suggest that having a child is a burning desire for everyone, nor do I presume that every woman feels a sensation of dread as her biological clock ticks past the age of fertility. But for those men and women who wish desperately to experience parenthood and haven't been able to, even being able to look forward to a future that holds some possibilities is a blessing.

Surrogate parenting is, and should remain, one of those possibilities. With an intelligent approach and conscientious guidance, the mechanics of a surrogate program could be established nationwide, thus eliminating some of the problems that now exist.

If it were not for the possibility of gestational surrogacy, two of my very precious children would not exist. But they do, and they are beautiful. Thanks to the compassion of two uniquely special women, Ness and Tanya could be born.

Genetic mother, surrogate womb, miracle baby. We have woven a delicate and loving web around each other, and we've touched each other's lives in an extremely profound way. The memory of these miraculous births, an incredible group effort, will stay with us for a lifetime.

I feel very strongly that the concept of surrogacy should thrive and, under proper guidance, be a positive possibility for those who battle infertility.

For many of us, it's nothing short of a miracle.

Feminists Should Support Surrogate Motherhood

by Laura M. Purdy

About the author: *Laura M. Purdy is an associate professor at Wells College in Aurora, New York. An expert in applied ethics, Purdy has published numerous articles on the ethical implications of reproductive technologies. She is the author of the book* In Their Best Interest? The Case Against Equal Rights for Children.

It is not surprising that the practice now widely known as "surrogate motherhood" has excited so much interest, so many articles, even books. The practice—even though it need involve nothing more high-tech than a turkey baster—invites us to reconsider some of the most fundamental human relationships and raises a host of issues and problems. What, if any, are the necessary and sufficient conditions of motherhood? Who should have the right to rear a child when biological mother and father do not live together? What are the grounds for claims to children, anyway? Is it wrong for women deliberately to bear a child for others to raise? And if not, should they be paid? The questions go on and on, and new twists like egg donation and contracted embryo gestation simply add more dimensions for moral philosophers and lawyers to ponder.

I have already argued elsewhere (and will not recapitulate the details here) that if stringently regulated with an eye toward women's welfare—a big "if"— contract pregnancy could offer significant benefits for them, and perhaps also for the babies. First, alleviating infertility can create much happiness for both women and men. Second, even where infertility is not the issue, there is often good reason to try to transfer burden or risk from one individual to another. Pregnancy may be a serious burden or risk for one woman, whereas it is much less so for another. Some women love being pregnant, others hate it; pregnancy interferes with work for some, but not others; pregnancy also poses much higher levels of risk to health (even life) for some than for others. Reducing burden and risk benefits not only the woman involved, but also the resulting

Excerpted from "Another Look at Contract Pregnancy" by Laura M. Purdy, in *Issues in Reproductive Technology: An Anthology*, edited by Helen Bequaert Holmes (New York: Garland Press, 1992). Reprinted by permission of the publisher.

child: high-risk pregnancies create, among other things, serious risk of prematurity, one of the major sources of handicap in babies. Society also benefits when expensive problems like prematurity are avoided. Furthermore, serious genetic diseases could be avoided by allowing some women to carry babies for others.

Third, contract pregnancy makes possible the creation of nontraditional families, which can be a significant source of happiness to single women and gay couples. Fourth, contract pregnancy could be the lowest technology method of achieving these

> *"'Surrogate motherhood'. . . invites us to reconsider some of the most fundamental human relationships."*

aims, uses the fewest medical resources, and could potentially be controlled mainly by women.

All these proposed advantages of contract pregnancy presuppose that there is some advantage in making possible at least partially genetically based relationships between parents and offspring. Although it is clear that we might be better off without this desire, I doubt that we will soon be free of it. This desire does not justify risking either women's or children's health; nobody's general well-being should be sacrificed to it, nor does it warrant huge social investments. However, it is something that, other things being equal, it would be good to satisfy as long as people continue to have anything like their current values.

Nevertheless, many objections to contract pregnancy have been raised. The transfer of risk and burden from one woman to another has been characterized as either contingently or necessarily involving class- or race-based exploitation. Another argument is that the practice degrades women because it reinforces the view of them as "brood-mares" and harms them by violating their maternal instincts. Furthermore, the practice is held to constitute morally undesirable baby selling, and to harm children by disrupting their sense of family. I believe that these objections are less well-founded than is generally recognized and have argued against them elsewhere. However, it also seems clear that there is more to be said about some of these issues. In particular, it would be helpful to look in more detail at ideals of motherhood, the moral status of infertility, and what I shall label "utilitarian worries."

Motherhood: Surrogate or Otherwise

One problematic aspect of the practice of women's bearing babies for others to rear, one that is indicative of the moral tangles lurking here, is what to call it. "Surrogate motherhood" seems inappropriate, both because it looks peculiar to call a woman pregnant with her own fertilized egg a surrogate and because it calls up undesirable associations with respect to motherhood. Sara Ann Ketchum attempted to resolve this problem by referring to the practice as "contracted motherhood" or "baby contracts." But the former creates similar assumptions about motherhood, while the latter seems to focus on the baby, leaving the woman invisible. Previously, I used "contracted pregnancy" which still seems to me the most accurate term; for simplicity's sake, I will shorten it to "contract pregnancy."

This is not just a semantic issue. Contract pregnancy (along with new conceptive technologies generally) raises pressing new questions about the whole notion of motherhood. Because language both expresses underlying assumptions and contributes to future ones, the implications of our linguistic choices are not always trivial.

> *"Contract pregnancy could offer significant benefits for [women], and perhaps also for the babies."*

My concern about calling pregnant women "mothers" is that it suggests without argument that they have at least the same obligations toward their fetuses that they do toward their children. That conclusion, however, should not be accepted without further argument, given its bearing both on the morality of abortion and on women's legal duties toward fetuses they plan to carry to term. A related problem, as Mary Mahowald notes, is that "mother" suggests fetuses are separate individuals, with all the moral baggage implied by that claim. It would therefore seem preferable to reserve the term "mother" for women who nurture a child.

This move seems perfectly plausible until we ask whose child she is nurturing. Does the child in question have to be biologically hers? If so, that leaves out many women who are doing all the same things mothers do. If not, then what is the status of the woman who bore the child? As the furor over the Baby M case shows, these issues should not be decided by manipulating definitions or by tradition—but by solid argument. In the meantime, neutral terms are needed that do not prejudice the matter one way or the other. It follows that Patricia Spallone's assertion that "the woman who goes through pregnancy and gives birth is the mother" is also to be regarded as problematic.

Splitting Biological and Social Relationships

Until recently such a claim would have been considered simply bizarre, for mothering just *was* the natural progression of pregnancy, labor, delivery, and nurturing. Of course, some unfortunate women and children did not fit this mold. Some women adopted children because they were unable to have their own; others married widowers or divorced men with children; still others got pregnant in inconvenient circumstances and gave up their babies for adoption. Likewise, some children lost their mothers and acquired "new" ones by dint of their fathers' remarriage or by being adopted. But these were peripheral cases— if not statistically, then psychologically. However, contemporary social conditions and scientific knowledge are, as Michelle Stanworth puts it, "deconstructing" motherhood: "motherhood as a unified biological process will be effectively deconstructed: in place of 'mother,' there will be ovarian mothers who supply eggs, uterine mothers who give birth to children and, presumably, social mothers who raise them."

What are we to make of this development? First, it constitutes explicit recognition of the split between biological and social relationships already existing in human lives. And, it should be noted that splitting the two has often enhanced welfare: it has, among other things, permitted women unable to rear their children to give them over to others more able to do so, a practice that has often benefitted all. Of course, too, the outcome has often been less satisfactory, as where adoptive parents have been insensitive to the special problems faced by their children, or where prejudice based on race, class or sexual orientation has led the state to appropriate children unjustifiably. Second, by now distinguishing genetic and gestational components of biological motherhood, deconstructed motherhood also constitutes a new dimension of that split.

The Image of Ideal Motherhood

This fragmentation of the concept "mother" is deeply disturbing to some critics of the new conceptive technologies, including many feminists. "Motherhood," is, after all, an enormously complicated term because of its emotional associations. They fear its loss and see it as a way of reducing women's power as mothers, just as the power inherent in skilled labor is undermined when complicated industrial processes are broken up into smaller sections, each of which can be done by more easily exploitable unskilled workers. In reproduction, the threat inherent in this process is reinforced by the fact that such a division of labor entails relying on technology controlled mainly by men: it takes technology to get eggs out of women, as well as to fertilize them and put them back in. Thus the division of labor and reliance on technology render the new conceptive technologies dangerous terrain for women.

That these worries constitute sufficient grounds for rejecting them seems to me dubious, although they do suggest a need for extreme caution. I am more troubled at present by something else. I am grateful to the radical feminist critics of the new conceptive practices for their vigorous attention to new developments, even though I often disagree with their conclusions, for they bring to light dimensions of the issues that might otherwise remain hidden. But their positions, too, sometimes rest on inadequately articulated presuppositions that need to be brought out into the open. In particular, I have

> *"Contract pregnancy makes possible the creation of nontraditional families."*

been increasingly concerned about the images of womanhood and motherhood upon which many of their criticisms of the conceptive technologies rest, images that draw much of their strength from a disconcerting appeal to nature that, as Stanworth argues, "ignores . . . the strenuous, and partly successful efforts of the women's movement to transcend the identification of women with nature."

The image I question is that of ideal motherhood, constituted by a natural progression of pregnancy, labor, and child rearing. . . .

Infertility and Its Remedies

The natural image of motherhood implicit in the comments of some feminist critics of the new technologies is integral to their conception of a new and better society. Yet this image seems to leave out in the cold women who cannot conceive when they want to. Nor does it leave any remedy for single individuals or homosexual couples. What about them? One thing seems clear: in that better society there will not be many—if any—babies available for adoption. Nor should there be any of the pitiful older children now desperate for good homes, the handicapped, the racially mixed, the emotionally disturbed; they will all be cared for already.

The radical feminist answer is, in part, as Patricia Spallone rightly points out, that infertility will be much reduced due to better "primary health care for women, screening for pelvic inflammatory disease and cervical cancer, by securing a higher standard of hygiene and nutrition for poor women, by cleaning up the workplace from environmental hazards that cause infertility in women and men, and congenital health problems in infants." One might also add that infertility could quite likely be reduced still further by social policies that permit women to have babies at a time in their life which is now "too soon" for many professions.

> *"For some people, their ties to children are the strongest and most enduring human connections they will ever make."*

What about those women who remain infertile despite all these improvements? Apparently, according to many radical feminists, they will have to grin and bear it: women do not really need babies to be fulfilled and their conviction that they do is just a consequence of socially promoted pronatalism. Yet this answer would not really be consistent with the more humane attitudes we all hope for in a better society, as that pronatalism would be gone, along with other patriarchal pressures. However, not only will there undoubtedly be a transitional period where the legacy of such pressures persists, but, more generally, the ease with which the desire for children is dismissed is troubling: I do not believe that the strong desire for children is merely an artifact of patriarchy. As a voluntarily childless woman myself, I am as aware as anybody that life can be fulfilling without a child of your own. However, as one who has also participated in parenting, I also know that—for better or worse—there is nothing else quite like it. It just will not do to tell people that they should adopt a Girl Scout troop instead. A special closeness arises from being a child's primary caretaker and a special thrill in witnessing the child's development into a human person. In addition, for some people, their ties to children are the strongest and most enduring human connections they will ever make. So long as we think human survival desirable, these interests are likely to unite into a wish to be involved in child rearing.

Now it is true that wanting X does not necessarily justify your having it; after all, going after it may be harmful to others so that their interests override yours. But rejecting women's desires as unreasonable or immoral without adequate consideration of possible compromises is a hallmark of traditional sexist attitudes toward women; it pains me to see it reproduced in some feminist thinking.

> *"Adoption is not necessarily the panacea it might seem."*

Unsympathetic Attitudes

A cavalier attitude toward the infertile, despite ritual expressions of concern for them, seems to me implicit in the answers currently promoted for infertile women who want children. They are told that their desire for a healthy, genetically related baby is not "authentic" and that if they truly want to be parents they should be ready to adopt an older child, even if he or she is handicapped, emotionally disturbed, or of a different ethnic background. It is also suggested that any attempt to create a new, genetically related child via conceptive technologies is so immoral as to override any standing the desire for such a child might have. These uncompromising and unsympathetic stands strike me as likely to obscure the important issues raised by radical feminist critiques.

Consider first that adoption is not necessarily the panacea it might seem. As Michelle Stanworth points out, "The description of infertility as a social condition of involuntary childlessness doesn't hold for all women. For some, pregnancy and childbirth are not only a route to a child, but a desired end in itself." This desire must surely count for something with those who want to validate women's experiences of gestation and labor.

She notes two other difficulties with adoption. First, "adoption and fostering are often subject to strict surveillance and regulation . . . not necessarily benign to women." She defends her claim by describing some of the standards used to judge whether women should be granted a child:

> Their policies and criteria of assessment are framed against a conventional notion of parenting—and particularly, of motherhood—which will deter many would-be mothers. Adoption agencies in Britain may (and often do) refuse single women or those aged over thirty; may (and usually do) refuse those who are not heterosexual, whether married or not; may (and sometimes do) refuse women who have jobs, women who have had psychiatric referrals, women with disabilities, women whose unconventional lifestyles cast doubt— for the social workers at least—on their suitability as mothers.

Second, adoption may well mean taking a child from another woman: "The pressures that lead some women to surrender their babies for adoption are very like those condemned in the case of surrogate mothers, right down to the possibility of exploitation of women from subordinate ethnic communities or from poorer nations." According to Stanworth, white parents in Britain can no longer easily adopt black children because of worry about the potential for exploitation of this sort. Such realism about the conditions and consequences of different remedies for problems like infertility is essential; all too often, the disadvantages of a disfavored solution are contrasted with the advantages of the favored one, where a more thorough assessment would suggest quite a different picture.

Even if a woman morally can adopt, reluctance to do so is often brushed off as prejudice by radical feminist critics of the new conceptive technologies. Thus, for instance, the desire for a young baby is, despite ample evidence of the importance of the early years for later development, discounted: infertile women should be ready to take on whatever painful legacy is left by inadequate care, just as they should be ready to take on the physical or emotional problems that might afflict a "hard-to-adopt" child.

A Problematic Position

As I have argued elsewhere, there are two points that need to be made about this position. On the one hand, raising difficult children is not a task to be undertaken lightly, for it can be so demanding as to require virtual abandonment of all other significant plans. It is easy for those who do not have to face such daily realities as high-priced, inaccessible medical care, incontinence, special equipment, full-time surveillance, lack of mobility, violent antisocial behavior, and the like to recommend that others should take them on. Nor should critics ignore the fact that, as society is currently organized, most of those left to cope with these problems will be women, not men. Is this the price radical feminists want to extract from their sisters who want to mother a child? "Normal" reproduction, too, is a kind of lottery, of course: fertile couples are not guaranteed normal children, although most get them. That some people are willing to devote their lives to difficult children is admirable and to be encouraged; asking those who might be excellent parents of a normal child to parent an especially demanding one may be, as things now stand, a recipe for misery and perhaps even child abuse. We, as a society, are not doing much to relieve such parents of the special burden they bear; providing this kind of help as a matter of course would undoubtedly also reduce the number of children given out for adoption as well as encourage adoption of those who are now given up. Our collective failure to render such help is unconscionable.

> *"Reasonable men . . . will not be precipitated by the existence of paid contract pregnancy to the view that women are primarily breeders."*

On the other hand, given our collective irresponsibility here, who are we to hold only the infertile responsible for difficult children? Why do we expect such supererogatory behavior of them without seeing that the same arguments apply to the fertile? Why, indeed, do radical feminists not argue that so long as there are homeless children, it is wrong for the *fertile* to have their own babies? As Stanworth rightly suggests, "Our critique of pronatalism and of reproductive technologies will be all the more persuasive when it ceases to distinguish so categorically between fertile women and infertile.". . .

> *"With respect to contract pregnancy no one has yet shown . . . [that] regulation is impossible."*

Utilitarian Worries

These points should make it clear that some objections to unorthodox reproduction are more problematic than they might at first seem. The ideal of motherhood against which practices like contract pregnancy are measured contains its own Achilles heel, and the most obvious traditional approaches to infertility may often be unsatisfactory. Contract pregnancy and other conceptive technologies might still not be justifiable, however, if radical feminists' conception of reality were accurate.

Some such feminists argue that men, as a class, and for a variety of reasons, want to control women. Women, despite a long history of restriction, still largely control reproduction, and much of their power and perceived value is predicated on this control. The new reproductive practices show promise, however, of finally putting reproduction in men's hands, partly because it is men who control technology and partly because technology has a logic of its own that promotes hierarchy. Hence, even if certain conceptive technologies benefit particular women, they harm women as a class.

The most extreme versions of this picture suggest that what men really want is to eliminate the need for women altogether. Now this aim would clearly be shortsighted, for we generally still do more than our share of such tasks as child rearing for which men in general show little enthusiasm. Furthermore, unless we are also to believe that all men are latent homosexuals, we would be missed in other ways as well.

But do men want to control (as opposed to eliminate) women? It is undeniable that some men do want to control us; it is also undeniable that many men unconsciously act in ways compatible with such a desire. If nothing else, the widespread violence against women shows that men's attitudes toward women are less than egalitarian. Women's inferior social position is obvious from the statistics on work, income, and wealth; that most positions of power are occupied by men also supports this conclusion.

Now this is obviously not the place for a detailed examination of the radical feminist view of society, but deciding about contract pregnancy cannot wait until that issue is resolved. How, in the meantime, is it possible to proceed?

First, it seems to me that the situation is a good deal more complicated than the foregoing would suggest. On the one hand, individual men do not necessarily hold these negative attitudes. On the other, factors like class and race interact with gender in ways that would complicate this picture considerably, even if it were accurate. Some writers, like Maria Mies, implicitly recognize this fact when they reject the claim that if and when more women become technical experts we would have less to fear from technology. For instance, she asserts that "we can no longer pursue the biologistic fallacy that social conditions would change if as many women as possible were sitting at the control panels of power, in the privileged positions in politics, economics, culture, and in the ever more elitist and centralist world of the new technology." She goes on to say that "we must ask what policies, what aims these women represent. The existing technology is still an instrument of domination if women control it. If they do not want to fight patriarchy and capital at the same time, they will turn it against women, too."

It will be no easy matter, given the ongoing and sometimes violent disagreement among feminists, to decide where this pessimistic view of human society intersects with reality. Despite the obvious hostility of substantial numbers of men, I am still unconvinced that the battle lines are so irrevocably drawn as the radical feminist picture would suggest. Furthermore, like Stanworth, I am convinced that even were it accurate, negativism about conceptive technologies is not necessarily the best coping strategy. She asks, for example, whether wholesale rejection of them

> *"The arguments against contract pregnancy do not show that it should be prohibited."*

> is really the best way to protect women who have sought (and will continue to seek) their use. An implacable opposition to conceptive technologies could mean that any chance of exerting pressure on those who organize infertility services—for example, pressure for better research and for disclosure of information; for more stringent conditions of consent; for means of access for poorer women, who are likely to be the majority of those with infertility problems—would be lost. Would it be wise to abandon infertile women to the untender mercies of infertility specialists, when a campaign, say, to limit the number of embryos that may be implanted (and thereby to reduce multiple pregnancies, pressures for selective reduction, and so forth), or to regulate the use of hormonal stimulation, might do a great deal to reduce the possible risks to women and to their infants?

Her general point, though well taken, still leaves unanswered the objection that it is not maltreatment of the infertile that is most worrisome, but the consequences for women as a group if the infertile, seeking to advance what they see as their own interest, make the overall situation worse. Among the objections of this type are that recourse to such practices as contract pregnancy, especially when money changes hands, promotes the view of women as breeders, exploits poor women, and is potentially racist in new and horrifying ways.

What evidence is there that letting women engage in contract pregnancies for money will cause deterioration in men's attitudes toward women? I believe that reasonable men who do not already have unfounded negative attitudes toward women will not be precipitated by the existence of paid contract pregnancy to the view that women are primarily breeders. However, we have little evidence one way or the other on this empirical issue; what *can* be said is that there is nothing about the practice itself that would justify any such judgment.

Surrogacy's Effect on Poor Women

Is the assertion that contract pregnancy exploits poor women better founded? I have shown elsewhere that arguments so far given for this claim are unsuccessful. Neither Christine Overall's Marxist argument that it constitutes an especially degrading kind of alienated labor nor the standard liberal argument about appropriate protection from risk are persuasive. The latter, in particular, depends upon ignorance of the kinds of risks working-class people routinely face; it also depends upon a refusal to take seriously the fact that circumstances ought to make a difference in whether a given act is judged prudent or moral.

What needs to be shown here is that contract pregnancy is more exploitive than other services the rich now buy from the poor. The rich, by definition, have more money than the poor; that is why the rich dine in expensive restaurants that employ poor waiters, hire help to clean their houses, and procure for themselves a variety of other services the poor cannot afford. Of course, the gap between rich and poor ought to be smaller so that the poor can have greater access to some of these luxuries. That way, for example, more poor women at risk for health problems in pregnancy could avoid them just as their richer sisters can now do via contract pregnancy. A more economically just society would not, by itself, necessarily provide women with appropriate protection from exploitation, although the pool of women who would submit to any indignity for money would be greatly reduced.

It is undeniable that the potential for exploitation in our own inegalitarian society is substantial, for poor women are much less able to protect their own interests than they would

> *"In a better society, the call for contract pregnancy would be less, but so would the risks."*

be in a better society. However, it does not follow from this that potentially exploitable but otherwise morally permissible practices should be banned altogether. One way to protect otherwise vulnerable individuals is to regulate them. With respect to contract pregnancy no one has yet shown either that it is not morally permissible or that such regulation is impossible. . . .

The arguments against contract pregnancy do not show that it should be prohibited; they do show that it must be stringently regulated so as to protect the interests of the women who participate. This would include standardized contracts guaranteeing the kind of conditions I have suggested here, such as better pay, physical autonomy, and so forth. Such a model contract would also have to contain clauses on other issues I have not argued for here, such as full pay for stillborn babies and perhaps provision for women (whether they provided their own egg or not) to change their mind about keeping the baby or having visitation rights. In the absence of such protections, women will be exploited and abused, and the practice should be discouraged or banned.

In general, I think that in a better society, the call for contract pregnancy would be less, but so would the risks. In our own society the practice could have, as I have argued, substantial benefits to all parties. It is tempting to reject such technological and social innovations out-of-hand, partly, perhaps, to counterbalance the uncritical enthusiasm with which every dream-child of science seems to be received in many quarters. It is also all too easy to evaluate them solely from our own privileged perspective, forgetting that it may blind us to the kinds of choices daily faced by some of those about whom we are arguing.

Surrogate Contracts Should Be Legalized

by Cherylon Robinson

About the author: *Cherylon Robinson is an assistant professor of sociology at the University of Texas at San Antonio.*

The legal structure partially defines roles within the family through state statutes dealing with marriage, divorce and parent-child relationships. The traditional legal definition of mother reflects the state's emphasis on the mother-fetus relationship. State statutes prescribe that the woman who gives birth to a child is considered to be the mother of the child. This definition was legislated partially because of the ease with which the mother's relationship to the child could be established; however, it also reflected an assumption that the components of the status, "mother," i.e., genetic, gestational, and social mothering, were connected. The legal definition of father, by declaring the husband of the mother the father of the child, reflects the male's relationship to the mother, not necessarily to the child. State statutes then partially define the roles of mother and father by defining the rights and responsibilities of the parents toward the child.

However, parenting roles in the United States are changing and, with those changes, both the mother-child relationship and the father-child relationship are being redefined. State statutes prescribe situations in which these rights and responsibilities of parents may be abdicated, such as in adoption. By allowing a birth mother to relinquish her rights and responsibilities toward her child and by accepting the transferral of rights and responsibilities to an adopting mother, the legal structure recognizes that the components of mothering could be separated and accomplished by different persons. Recent medical technologies have complicated the issue of defining the mother of a child by making it possible for components of the status, mother, to be accomplished by three different people (a genetic mother, a gestational mother, and a social mother). This possibility requires that the relative importance of these three components in our notion of "who is a mother?" be examined. . . .

Excerpted from "Surrogate Motherhood: Implications for the Mother-Fetus Relationship" by Cherylon Robinson, in *The Politics of Pregnancy: Policy Dilemmas in the Maternal-Fetal Relationship*, edited by Janna C. Merrick and Robert H. Blank (Binghamton, NY: Haworth Press, 1993); ©1993 by The Haworth Press, Inc. Reprinted with permission.

Reproductive technology involves the use of medical technology to achieve asexual reproduction and has included artificial insemination, in vitro fertilization, cryopreservation of ova, sperm and embryos, embryo transfer and the use of these procedures for surrogate motherhood arrangements. Surrogate motherhood arrangements involve the agreement of the surrogate to conceive through the use of reproductive technology, to gestate the fetus conceived and then give up the child at birth to his/her genetic father and/or genetic mother. Artificial insemination of a surrogate with the semen of the man intended to be the father is the most common procedure utilized in surrogate motherhood; however, embryo lavage or embryo transfer may be used to achieve surrogate gestation. Surrogate gestation involves the gestation of a fetus genetically unrelated to the surrogate.

> *"Surrogate motherhood provides a reproductive alternative to childlessness and/or adoption."*

These different technologies provide the possibility for infertile couples to reproduce, a possibility that sometimes gets minimized in the debate over their usage. The grief of infertile couples is real, and the attraction of being able to have a child which is genetically related to one or both parent(s) is strong. However, debate over the legitimation of different reproductive technologies has raised complex societal, legal and ethical issues related to their usage. One of those issues involves the potential for reproductive technology to redefine the concept, mother, and subsequently decrease the saliency of the gestational role in that definition, thus altering the mother-fetus relationship. This issue is especially important in the debate over legitimation of surrogate motherhood because surrogates are required to relinquish their parental rights and responsibilities. . . .

The Legal Status

Few states have passed statutes that specifically deal with surrogate motherhood (see Table 1). Additionally, state statutes that do exist are not consistent in their recognition of, or prohibition of, surrogate motherhood arrangements. Ten states have passed laws that would prohibit commercial surrogate motherhood arrangements. Three states have passed laws that legitimate noncommercial surrogate motherhood arrangements but would prohibit compensation in these arrangements. A third state possibly permits both commercial and noncommercial surrogacy arrangements. It is unclear whether existing laws passed to define parent-child relationships in other situations, such as adoption and artificial insemination by donor, are applicable to surrogacy. At least five states exclude surrogate motherhood from existing statutes on adoption or artificial insemination. These statutes would prevent prohibition of surrogate motherhood based on existing statutes.

In court decisions on the applicability of statutes dealing with adoption and

Table 1. Surrogate Motherhood Statutes

Statutes	Noncommercial Surrogate Motherhood Legitimated	Commercial Surrogate Motherhood Legitimated
Arizona	no	no
Arkansas	yes	unclear
Florida	yes	no
Indiana	no	no
Kentucky	no	no
Louisiana	no	no
Michigan	no	no
Nebraska	no	no
New Hampshire	yes	no
New York	no	no
North Dakota	no	no
Utah	no	no
Virginia	yes	no
Washington	no	no

artificial insemination to surrogate motherhood, opinions have been mixed as well. Some court cases have held that surrogate motherhood does violate state statutes, and others have ruled that it does not. In states where surrogate motherhood is prohibited or not excluded from existing statutes, the contract is probably unenforceable in most states. . . .

A Legal Lag

The legal structure plays a significant role in defining the normative structure within which the family operates. State statutes define who is to be considered the mother and who is to be considered the father of a child and what rights and responsibilities are associated with these relationships. Surrogate motherhood provides a reproductive alternative to childlessness and/or adoption that is attractive to many individuals. For this reason, surrogate motherhood arrangements will probably continue to be made whether or not they are legitimated by the legal system. If these arrangements are made without legitimation, they will be made in an unregulated manner that could have serious consequences. Unregulated surrogate motherhood arrangements have potential for generating conflict over the rights and responsibilities of the individuals toward the child.

At present a legal lag exists between the development of reproductive technology and the response of the legal structure to its use in surrogate motherhood arrangements. This legal lag has resulted in legal ambiguity related to the parenting rights and responsibilities of involved individuals. In the process of responding to this ambiguity and conflicts related to it through legislation or adjudication, the legal structure will define, or redefine, the concept, mother. This definition, or redefinition, will potentially impact on the mother-fetus relationship by increasing or decreasing its importance. At present, it appears that the limited legal response has decreased the importance of the gestational component of the definition of mother and thus decreased the importance of the relationship between the mother and the fetus.

Legitimation of surrogate motherhood would increase the saliency of the social role in the legal definition of mother. This definition places an emphasis on the importance of the fulfillment of the rights and responsibilities of the mother in the relationship between the mother and the child. It would also take into consideration an increased social recognition that rights and responsibilities of parenting, in-

> *"Unregulated surrogate motherhood arrangements have potential for generating conflict."*

cluding nurturing, may be accomplished by someone other than a biological parent, e.g., a stepparent, regardless of gender. The responsibility of nurturing, for example, is increasingly becoming part of our notion of the responsibilities of fathers. Thus, legal emphasis on the social role in the mother-child relationship as a social role reflecting intentions, rights and responsibilities but not necessarily a gestational relationship would be compatible with the social changes that have already occurred in the United States.

An increased emphasis on the genetic role in defining the mother-child relationship would also be consistent with legal and social changes. Advances in medical technology have increased our ability to define genetic links between individuals. The historical notion of defining a father-child relationship by the male's relationship to the mother has been undermined by statutes that allow rebuttal of paternity through the use of these medical advances.

Personal Liberties vs. State Interests

If legitimation of surrogate motherhood is extended further in the legal structure, it will very likely take some form of contractual parenting. Further consideration of legitimation of surrogate motherhood through legislation proposals, however, should address specific questions that consider the possible conflict between personal liberties and compelling state interests.

- Should remuneration for surrogates be allowed? If so, what would be appropriate remuneration? Or does remuneration violate compelling state interests prohibiting exploitation of poor women and/or commercialization of reproduction?
- Should surrogate motherhood be utilized only by infertile couples? Would utilization by singles, homosexual couples, or other alternatives to the nuclear family violate a compelling state interest in protection of the family?

- Under what circumstances and for how long should the parties involved be allowed to void the contract? Would prohibiting a surrogate from breaching the contract by failing to terminate parental rights violate a compelling state interest in protection of the mother-child relationship?
- Who should control the conduct of the surrogate during pregnancy: the surrogate, the physician, the couple? Could the surrogate's right to autonomy in pregnancy decisions be undermined by recognition of the rights of the fetus as a full human being?

Debate on these questions, however, should include views other than those of the legal structure and should take into consideration the societal, political and economic impact of legitimation. If surrogate motherhood is legitimated and regulated, there will be a potential for societal consequences that have not been anticipated. One of the unintended consequences of legitimated surrogate motherhood could involve a decrease in the perceived importance of gestation in the definition of mother and an increased emphasis on the genetic and social roles in this definition. Contractual parenting requires that the intentions, rights and responsibilities of all parties involved be delineated in the contract. This procedure calls for the introduction of rationality into an area of social life which is laden with emotion. This extension of rationality represents a departure from traditional notions on the importance of the mother-fetus relationship. Contracting to relinquish parental rights by the gestational mother is a major part of this departure. Indeed, this may be the most disturbing aspect of surrogate motherhood for many people. Others, however, may view this aspect of surrogate motherhood as very positive. Through contractual parenting in surrogate motherhood, each child would be conceived intentionally by individuals who want that child very much and would, therefore, presumably be conscientious in their fulfillment of the responsibilities defined by the parent/child relationship.

> *"Legitimation of surrogate motherhood would increase the saliency of the social role in the legal definition of mother."*

Surrogate Motherhood Harms Women

by Robyn Rowland

About the author: *Robyn Rowland is a social psychologist and senior lecturer in women's studies at Deakin University in Geelong, Victoria, Australia. She has contributed to the books* Test-Tube Women: What Future for Motherhood? *and* Man-Made Women: How Reproductive Technology Affects Women *and is the author of the book* Living Laboratories: Women and Reproductive Technologies, *from which this viewpoint is excerpted.*

> One woman in Texas was working full time, was recovering from a recent divorce which had created considerable debt, and was the type of person who was always willing to lend a helping hand. Surrogate motherhood, advertised in a supermarket tabloid, seemed like the perfect solution. Unfortunately, her heart condition was not discovered by her doctor until her sixth month of pregnancy. In spite of her pleading with a cardiologist to find the cause of her rapid heartbeat and shortness of breath, her appeal for help was never taken seriously. She did not have two hundred and fifty dollars for the heart monitor her doctor told her to wear; the baby broker never offered assistance; and in her eighth month of pregnancy, less than four weeks from the expected birth of the child she had nicknamed Jackie, Denise was found dead in her bed with her unborn son nestled inside her. . . . Her mother Pat is a friend of mine. . . . Pat was the one who received the bodies of her daughter and her grandson to bury on her farm. She never heard a word from the baby broker, or the sperm donor and his wife.

So writes Elizabeth Kane, the first commercial 'surrogate' in the US, a birth mother now active in the National Coalition Against Surrogacy, a woman who said she felt like a 'flesh-covered test-tube' during the experience. As the fetus becomes personalised, women are presented as less like people, they are dismembered and fragmented. They become eggs, ovaries, wombs, body parts disconnected from the whole person—merely vehicles for breeding babies. . . . The term 'surrogate mother' reinforces this picture. 'Surrogate' means 'substitute' (not a *real* mother), yet the woman is actually the *birth mother* and has a relationship with the child born based on the intimacy of its development inside her body and the relationship she has formed with the fetus and with the imagined child. Men tend to negate this experience, make it invisible and unimportant, because it is so unfamiliar to them.

Some 'surrogacy' arrangements take place with what is called, coyly, 'natural insemination by donor'. In its final report the Waller Committee in Victoria, Australia, said it had been told of a number of cases where women had had sexual intercourse with the fertile husbands of infertile women. The children born from these relationships had been handed to the father when they were born. Both Kirsty Stevens (UK) and 'Jane Smith', an Australian surrogate, produced their children through sexual intercourse.

High-Tech Surrogacy

But 'surrogacy' is more often connected with reproductive and birth technologies. It has moved away from the bedroom and into the laboratory through the use of artificial insemination by donor, or more frequently procedures such as IVF and sex determination. In the USA Patricia Foster underwent sex-determination procedures because the sperm donor wanted to have a son. Mary Beth Whitehead was coerced into undergoing amniocentesis and pre-natal diagnosis though it was unlikely that she would need it. Shannon Boff was involved in a surrogacy case with in vitro fertilisation using a donor egg. The egg was extracted from the infertile woman, fertilised in the laboratory with the husband's sperm and then transferred to Boff's womb. Cases involving the superovulation of women (breeders), using drugs which . . . may be potentially dangerous, have also occurred.

Nancy Barrass was prescribed Clomid. She was deliberately inseminated with sperm which both the doctor and the biological father knew to be contaminated with a bacterial infection. She was prescribed antibiotics for the infection she developed, as well as Clomid, which resulted in a cyst on her ovary. It seems that she was prescribed Clomid because the infection might make pregnancy difficult to attain. But they did not wait for the infection to be cured, 'he prescribed a triple dose of Clomid and continued to inseminate me'. She suffered unpleasant side effects. 'I experienced dizziness, blurred vision, a severe facial rash and intense pain in my left ovary. I was unable to walk because of the pain'.

> *"Elizabeth Kane . . . felt like a 'flesh-covered test-tube' during the experience."*

This triple mix of IVF, the donor egg and superovulation drugs was also used on South African Pat Anthony, who gave birth to triplets for her daughter, Karen (the children were referred to as her grandchildren). Karen was superovulated to produce the eleven eggs from which the embryos formed and was given hormones to enable her to breastfeed. In the Australian case of one sister bearing a child for another, the infertile sister was superovulated.

Contracting Women to Breed

So-called surrogacy takes place in various ways: through commercial agencies; through independent arrangements, often contractual, with money changing hands; and between friends or family members, often using IVF and an egg donated by the woman intending to raise the child.

Some states in the US, Indiana and Nebraska for example, are dealing with commercial 'surrogacy' by making contracts unenforceable in their courts. In the UK it is now illegal, as it is in the Australian states of Victoria, South Australia, Queensland and Western Australia. Nevertheless, contracts are made. Money may not change hands, but when a woman agrees to carry a child and hand it to another person at birth, she is contracting her body and herself.

The contracting man usually wants control over the type of woman who is to bear the child. This control is enshrined within the contracts. In a shocking exposé of these contracts in the US Susan Ince writes that she was expected to refrain from any sexual relations; refrain from smoking and drinking; keep all appointments whether medical, psychological and legal determined by the agency; use only those services provided by the agency; and undergo any medical treatment specified by the 'buyer' or agent. She had to abort if the fetus was abnormal, and if she willingly aborted a normal fetus or refused to relinquish the child the fa-

> *"The financial exploitation of women through surrogacy reinforces power differentials between classes of women."*

ther could sue her for the $25,000 he paid, plus costs. Both the buyer and the 'breeder' signed a clause saying that 'no matter what happens the company is not responsible'. Emphasis was placed on the woman being 'obedient', and Ince's minimal questioning of the contract was labelled 'selfish' and 'dangerous'. Clauses requiring genetic tests on the fetus allowed for the possibility of abortion if the sex of the child were 'wrong'. Similar controls were placed on Kim Cotton in the UK (before legislation banning commercial surrogacy was enacted in 1985) and on other American 'surrogates'.

An 'Alternative Reproduction Vehicle'

In the Mary Beth Whitehead case in the US the contract laid down that Whitehead would not abort unless her health was at risk, but must do so if Stern (the sperm donor) required it, and that she would undergo amniocentesis if he demanded it. She agreed not to smoke, drink alcohol, or use illegal, prescription or non-prescribed medications without the *written* consent of a doctor. Ironically, in order to ensure that Whitehead's husband, Richard, could not be declared the legal father of the child (which was conceived through artificial insemination), he had to sign a clause where he 'expressed his refusal to consent to the insemination of Mary Beth Whitehead'. Thus full and total responsibility falls on the woman. Finally,

> Mary Beth Whitehead, surrogate, and Richard Whitehead, her husband, understand and agree to assume all risks, including the risk of death, which are incidental to conception, pregnancy and childbirth, including but not limited to, post partum complications. [The Stern/Whitehead contract, as cited in an article by Rita Arditti.]

Whitehead took extreme means to avoid having to relinquish her child, but she and Stern ended up in the Superior Court of New Jersey under Judge Harvey Sorkow. Sorkow pilloried Whitehead's character and behaviour as a wife and mother. He accused her

> *"Childbearing for another is underpaid and undervalued."*

of being sly and of using her children to gain publicity. He implied that she would not be able to educate her children adequately because she herself was not educated. He compared her unfavourably to the Sterns, including Mrs Stern who was a paediatrician but who would 'not work full-time because she is aware of the infant's needs that will require her presence'. Sorkow ruled that Whitehead was 'manipulative, impulsive and exploitive' as well as 'untruthful'. He awarded custody to the 'father', in an outrageous statement which placed the birth mother in the same category as a prostitute. In Sorkow's words:

> The fact is, however, that the money to be paid to the surrogate is not being paid for the surrender of the child to the father. And that is just the point—at birth, mother and father have equal rights to the child absent [*sic*] any other agreement. The biological father pays the surrogate for her willingness to be impregnated and carry his child to term. At birth, the father does not purchase the child. It is his own biological genetically related child. He cannot purchase what is already his . . . this Court therefore will specifically enforce the surrogate parenting agreement to *compel* delivery of the child to the father and to terminate the mother's parental rights.

So the child belongs to the sperm donor but the mother is merely, in Sorkow's words, 'this alternative reproduction vehicle'. On 3 February 1988, however, the New Jersey Supreme Court ruled that commercial surrogate motherhood contracts were illegal, and Mary Beth Whitehead gained parental rights. All aspects of the Sorkow decision were overturned in a 7-0 ruling, except for custody which remained with Stern and his wife.

Disillusionment with Surrogacy

Despite this partial victory, the outcome was not a happy one for Mary Beth Whitehead. It is also not a happy one for other 'surrogates' who are still fighting their cases in various states. Elizabeth Kane still does not have custody of her child. Patricia Foster does not have custody of her child. . . .

Chapter 3

Paying Women to Be Surrogates

The financial exploitation of women through surrogacy reinforces power differentials between classes of women. Money is not the only motivating factor, but for many it is a crucial element. In one study of 125 women who wanted to be surrogate mothers, Philip J. Parker found that 40 per cent were unemployed at the time of interview or in need of financial aid. Their family income was not high and they did not generally have a high level of education. Surrogates are often uneducated, seeking a better education for their children.

Few women go through the surrogacy process for nothing. When Noel Keane, a lawyer with a large clientele in the US, advertised for surrogates but could not pay them under Michigan law, 'the numbers of volunteers dropped to almost zero'. Payment of 'surrogates' in the US seems to have remained for some years around $10 000–12 000 for what may be a two-year period of work, including pre-selection screening, a number of attempts at insemination, and the pregnancy and birth. William Handel of the Surrogate Parent Foundation, visiting Australia to investigate the establishment of such companies, said he paid surrogates this amount and paid himself $6000 per surrogate for what he described as 'an extraordinary amount of work on his part'.

> *"It is often during the pregnancy that women come to regret their decision."*

In England, an American surrogacy agent, Harriet Blankfield, was hiring Irish, Scottish and English breeders for £6500 [about $9900 US]. Because the babies left the country, the possibility of interference from the mother was reduced. An interesting comparison can be made here with sperm donors' rates of pay at the time. In England men were paid £7 [about $11 US] per half hour. If this extended to twenty-four hours a day for a nine-month pregnancy, Kim Cotton, Britain's most notable commercial 'surrogate', should have been paid around £90 000 [about $137,000 US]. Like other work women do, childbearing for another is underpaid and undervalued.

John Stehura, President of the Bioethics Foundation Inc., has said that he intends the fee to become smaller as surrogacy becomes more commonplace and as he gains more women from poorer parts of the US to add to his list. Dr Howard Adelman, who was screening women for Surrogate Mothering Ltd, feels that women in financial need are the 'safest' because if the woman is on unemployment and has a child to care for, 'she is not likely to change her mind'. This economic exploitation of women seems not to worry ethicists in Australia like Alan Rassaby, who wrote that 'given a choice between poverty and exploitation, many people [women?] may prefer the latter'. Calling these alternatives 'choices' makes a mockery of the term. The attitude condones the increasing pauperisation of women. . . .

Commercial companies spend time and effort 'counselling' women to convince them that the children they give birth to are not theirs. The women also

100

expend considerable emotional energy convincing themselves of the same thing. Pat Anthony said, 'I was only the incubator for them to grow in'; Mary Stewart, a Scottish single mother, wrote, 'I was just like a postie delivering the mail', and Australian 'Jane Smith' said, 'I don't think of the baby as mine. The way I see it I'm just a chook sitting on their nest until the eggs are ready to hatch'. Other women recognise the deception and self-deception involved in this objec-

> *"Surrogate motherhood is nothing more than the transference of pain from one woman to another."*

tification: 'I used to call myself a human incubator. I truly believed that what I was doing was more medical than emotional', wrote Elizabeth Kane. As Mary Beth Whitehead wrote:

> I remember the inseminating doctor telling me that I was giving away an egg.
> I didn't give away an egg. They took a baby away from me, not an egg. That
> was my daughter. That was Sara they took from me.

It is often during the pregnancy that women come to regret their decision, particularly after the baby has moved. Australian surrogate 'Jane Smith' said that at five months she had a scan and watched the baby move, 'And I suppose that did it. Before, I had somehow convinced myself that this wasn't "my" baby'. Mary Beth Whitehead says, 'It wasn't until the day I delivered her that I finally understood that I wasn't giving Betsy Stern her baby. I was giving her *my* baby'. Patricia Foster wrote of 'praying not to go into labour so you and the baby can't be separated'. . . .

Elizabeth Kane maintains that 'surrogate motherhood is nothing more than the transference of pain from one woman to another', and Patricia Foster writes, 'Infertile women sometimes say they feel pain every time they see a baby, a child. I'm the one who now looks at every child that goes by, at every crying baby that I hear, to check if it is my child'.

So-called surrogate motherhood is creating our next generation of grieving women.

Feminists Should Oppose Surrogate Motherhood

by Janice G. Raymond

About the author: *Janice G. Raymond is professor of women's studies and medical ethics at the University of Massachusetts, Amherst. She lectures internationally on reproductive and genetic technologies, feminist theory, and bioethics. Her books include* A Passion for Friends, The Transsexual Empire, *the coauthored* RU 486: Misconceptions, Myths and Morals, *and* Women as Wombs: Reproductive Technologies and the Battle over Women's Freedom, *from which this viewpoint is excerpted.*

When I was in graduate school, one of my medical ethics professors asserted that technological reproduction was "at least half a century off." That was 1971; this is 1993. "Half a century off" was also the public's forecast for the advent of reproductive and genetic technologies until scientists publicized their first documented in vitro fertilization (IVF) achievement in 1978. Baby Louise Brown became the world's first technological child, and the planet was put on notice that the technological was made flesh. . . .

A Question of Choice and Reproductive Rights?

New reproductive arrangements are presented as a woman's private choice. But they are publicly sanctioned violence against women. The absoluteness of this privatized perspective, especially as emphasized by the medical profession and the media, who present women as having unconditioned free will, functions as a smoke screen for medical experimentation and, ultimately, for the violation of women's bodies. Choice so dominates the discourse that it is almost impossible to recognize the injury that is done to women.

Choice resonates as a quintessential U.S. value set in the context of a social history that has gradually allowed all sorts of oppressive so-called options, such as prostitution, pornography, and breast implants, to be defended in the name of women's right to choose. The language of choice is compelling because it highlights a freedom that many women seldom have and a cafeteria of options disguised as self-determination. Viewing reproductive technologies and contracts mainly as a woman's choice results from a particular Western ideology that emphasizes individual freedom and value neutrality. At the same time, this ideology prevents us from examining technological and contractual reproduction as an institution and leads us to neglect the conditions that create industrialized breeding and the role that it plays in society. Choice so dominates the discussion that when critics of technological reproduction denounce the ways in which women are abused by these procedures, we are accused of making women into victims and, supposedly, of denying that women are capable of choice. To expose the victimization of women is to be blamed for creating women as victims.

> *"Surrogate contracts are outright constraints on women's capacity to choose."*

Whose interests are served by representing technological reproduction as a woman's private choice while rendering invisible the force of institutionalized male-dominant interests? Furthermore, is choice the real issue, or is the issue *what* those choices are and in what context selective women's choices (surrogacy or IVF) are fostered? At the very least, choice implies awareness of possible consequences—what women lack in the reproductive technological and contractual context. At the very most, choice implies that women's health, autonomy, integrity, and basic social justice are served.

Various reproductive rights groups have included within their list of demands access to technological reproduction and surrogacy. Technological reproduction is sometimes defended as part of the pro-choice platform. Borrowing from the abortion defense, reproductive liberals contend that feminists must support these technologies and contracts as part of a woman's right to choose. The right to abortion is combined with the right to reproductive technologies and contracts as a total package that many women feel compelled to accept.

No Real "Choice"

In the supposed interests of women, reproductive liberals have tried to silence critics of technological and contractual reproduction with the accusation that if we speak out against these procedures, we endanger women's reproductive freedom and give arguments to the anti-abortionists. Every criticism of these procedures is linked with the foes of abortion and subjected to the charges of stifling technology, freedom of research, and repressing women's choice. There is a vast difference, however, between women's right to choose safe, legal abortions and women's right to choose unsafe, experimental, and demeaning technologies and contracts. One allows genuine control over the course of a life; the other promotes abdication of control over the self, the body, and reproduction in general. Furthermore, our response to the right wing cannot simply be, "babies made to order." The concept of choice, if it is to have any feminist value, must not be advanced as an absolute right, else it risks reduction to a mere market consumerism.

The subverting of choice by the medical and corporate professionals to promote technological and contractual reproduction has been a largely unexamined area. The rhetoric of choice, however, belies its reality for women. Often what gets promoted as choice, such as the right to choose surrogate contracts, are outright constraints on women's capacity to choose. We cannot continue to pay lip service to reproductive choice while totally ignoring the control that these reproductive arrangements exercise over women.

Focus on the Fetus

I contend that those who *support* and *promote* technological and contractual reproduction are *undermining* women's reproductive rights, especially women's right to abortion. The extent to which the rights of women are diminished when the fetus is part of the woman's body—for example, in conservative anti-abortion policy and legislation—should make us seriously question the extent to which they will be further diminished as the fetus is increasingly removed from the female body. Whether in the womb or outside, attention is riveted on the fetus as individual entity—patient, person, or experimentee. IVF; embryo experimentation, transfer, and freezing; and fetal tissue research sever the embryo/ fetus from the woman. Reproductive technologies and contracts augment the rights of fetuses and would-be fathers while challenging the one right that women have historically retained some vestige of—mother-right.

> *"Those who* support *and* promote . . . *contractual reproduction are* undermining *women's reproductive rights."*

We witness this assault on women's rights in surrogate custody disputes and in frozen embryo contests where the rights of "ejaculatory fathers" are presented as men's rights to gender equality (or, as the fathers' rights movement phrases it, "Equal rights are not for women only"). These techniques render women as spectators of rather than participants in the whole reproductive process. More and more, they reduce women to the status of vehicle for the fetus; biologically, they literally sunder the fetus from the pregnant woman. Politically and legally, technological reproduction tends to position the fetus as isolated and independent from the mother but not from the sperm source, the doctor, or the state. . . .

Women as Victims

The social and political construction of female reality is a basic tenet of modern feminism. The feminist saying, "the personal is political," reveals that women's choices have not only been socially but politically orchestrated as well. When men and women act in certain ways, they are more than mere products of their socialization. Social conditioning theories often lack a political framework. Male domination and female subordination are bound up with power. There are positive advantages in status, ego, and authority for men in the ways, for example, they exercise their sexuality. The male power modes of sexuality construct women's sexual and reproductive lives to conform to male dictates.

> *"In surrogate agencies, there is a conjunction of male medical, corporate, and legal interests promoting the reproductive management of women."*

When radical feminists stress how women's reproductive choices are influenced by the social and political system and how women are channeled into having children at any cost to themselves, we are reproached for portraying women as victims. These reproaches have come mainly from feminist liberals but, increasingly, they are being echoed by liberal men. In the Baby M case [in which surrogate mother Mary Beth Whitehead attempted to keep the baby, and was ultimately given visitation rights], Gary Skoloff, the lawyer for Bill Stern, summed up his court argument by stating, "If you prevent women from becoming surrogate mothers . . . you are saying that they do not have the ability to make their own decisions. . . . It's being unfairly paternalistic and it's an insult to the female population of this nation." Skoloff probably learned this lingo from liberal lawyer Lori Andrews, who wrote, "Great care needs to be taken not to portray women as incapable of responsible decisions."

Choice occurs in the context of a society where, to put it mildly, there are fundamental differences of power between men and women. Yet feminists who oppose technological and contractual reproduction are vilified for supposedly claiming that "infertile women and, by implication, all women [are] incapable of rationally grounded and authentic choice," as stated by Michelle Stanworth. Little is said about why women are willing to submit their bodies to the most invasive and harmful medical interventions—for example, because their lives are devalued without children, because of husband/family pressure, because there has been little research and few resources devoted to infertility, and because women are channeled into abusive technologies at any cost to themselves. There is the presumption that if women choose to treat their bodies in this way—as reproductive experiments, vehicles, or objects for another's use—this is not problematic. This argument *is* problematic, however, because it minimizes the social and political contexts in which women's choices are made. Even the New Jersey Supreme Court decision, *In the Matter of Baby M*, recognized that although many women make a choice to enter surrogate arrangements and many others do not perceive surrogacy as exploitative, this "does not diminish its potential for devaluation to other women."

In addition to surrogacy and the new reproductive technologies, sexual and reproductive liberals have also claimed that women freely choose to enter pornography. This idea of pornography as a woman's unadulterated choice appeared most prominently in a document called the FACT (Feminist Anti-Censorship Taskforce) Brief. FACT organized for the sole purpose of defeating the Andrea Dworkin–Catharine MacKinnon feminist antipornography ordinance that makes pornography legally actionable as a violation of women's civil rights. Throughout the FACT Brief, the rhetoric of false victimization prevails. "The ordinance . . . reinforces sexist images of women as incapable of consent. . . . In effect, the ordinance creates a strong presumption that women who participate in the creation of sexually explicit material [FACT's euphemism for pornography] are coerced." The FACT Brief went so far as to say that women have been stereotyped as victims by the statutory rape laws.

Radical feminists stress how male supremacy channels women into pornography and surrogacy as well as into other reproductive procedures, while liberals charge that radical feminists make women into victims. There is a mechanism of denial operating in these accusations. In saying that women are not victims of male dominance, the liberal critics absolve themselves of responsibility for the victims. They obscure the necessity to create social and political change for those who are victims and they disidentify with their own victimization.

> *"Many women who have been victims of . . . surrogacy have become the system's most powerful critics."*

The kind of choice that feminist critics of technological and contractual reproduction would defend is substantive, not a so-called woman's choice growing out of a context of powerlessness. Instead, the more substantive question is, Do such so-called choices as surrogacy foster the empowerment of women as a group and create a better world for women? What kind of choices do women have when subordination, poverty, and degrading work are the options available to many? The point is not to deny that women are capable of choosing within contexts of powerlessness, but to question how much real value, worth, and power these so-called choices have.

Women make choices about what they judge to be in their own self-interest or survival, often in a desperate attempt to find safety or security, and often to give meaning to their existence. Andrea Dworkin, in *Right-Wing Women*, demonstrates that politically conservative as well as feminist women are aware of the ways in which women are subordinated to male dictates, yet the former make different choices than feminists do. They choose what they perceive to be in their own best interests. Like most women, they make survival choices in a context of restricted options. So are we then to anoint their choices merely because they freely choose? In a similar way, *because* some women choose to enter surrogate contracts or submit themselves to the bodily invasions of multiple IVF treatments does not validate those choices.

In one way, this discussion of the social and political construction of women's choices demonstrates the old philosophical debate between freedom and necessity. Necessity is imposed through the social forces that dictate the conditions of women's lives, conditions that women do not create. That women do not often create the social conditions within which they act does not abrogate their capacity to choose, but it does call for a more complex assessment of what we call women's choices, bidding us to focus less on choice and more on its constraints. What are the organized forces shaping women's choice of surrogacy and other reproductive techniques? For starters, the whole social context of sexual subordination in which women live their lives and which results, for many, in economic poverty, dead-ended jobs, and low self-esteem. In surrogate agencies, there is a conjunction of male medical, corporate, and legal interests promoting the reproductive management of women. The media put on a promotional show, as well.

Victims, but Not Passive

This is not to say that women who sign surrogate contracts are *simply* passive victims. Women's victimization can be acknowledged without labeling women passive. *Passive* and *victim* do not necessarily go together. Jews were victims of the Nazis, but they were not passive, nor did the reality of victimization define the totality of their existence. Blacks were victims of slavery, yet no thoughtful commentator would ever portray slaves as passive. It seems obvious that women can be victims of pornography and technological reproduction without depriving women of some ability to act under oppressive conditions, else how could any woman extract herself from these conditions, as many have?

Feminists can move beyond a one-dimensional focus on women's oppression without relinquishing the critique of women's oppression. This is the most serious failure of sexual and reproductive liberalism—*the relinquishing of the critique of the oppression of women.* The end result of this abdication is that while lip service may be paid in minimal ways to the "possible" abuses of surrogacy and the new reproductive technologies, the present ways in which women do move beyond sexual and reproductive violence are never validated. For example, the sexual and reproductive liberal literature does not mention the exsurrogates and the expornography models who have organized to fight against surrogacy and pornography instead of promoting these as economic options for women. Many women who have been victims of pornography and surrogacy have become the systems' most powerful critics, but we are, instead, urged to examine the ways in which these systems of pornography and surrogacy, for example, are useful to women.

> *"When pornography and surrogacy are idealized as choices, this defines a new range of conformity for women."*

Finally, it seems obvious that one can recognize women's victimization by these institutions without shoring up the institutions themselves. When the sexual and reproductive liberals affirm that women are agents in a "culture" of pornography and technological reproduction, they sideline the agency of the institutions, thereby letting them off the hook. Why find evidence of women's agency *within* institutions of women's oppression and then use that agency to bolster these very systems? Why not locate women's agency in resistance to these institutions—for example, the agency of women who have courageously testified about their abuse in pornography and surrogacy, risking

> *"Women are left with the hollow rhetoric of choice— in reality, no choice at all."*

exposure and ridicule and often getting it; the exsurrogates who have fought for themselves and their children in court against the far greater advantages of the sperm source. Why locate women's agency primarily within the "culture" of male supremacy? And why shift attention from an analysis and activism aimed at destroying these systems to a justification of them? By romanticizing the victimization of women as liberating, sexual and reproductive liberalism leaves women in these systems at the mercy of them.

Sexual and reproductive liberalism has produced a new idealization of women's oppression; it defends the institution of surrogacy as providing the means for women's economic survival and the institution of pornography as freeing the expression of a repressed outlaw female sexuality. This idealization makes women's subordination and abuse honorable, much in the tradition of the nineteenth-century view of ennobling women's domestic confinement and "conservation of energy." If oppression produces sexually or reproductively "free" women, it is a grand case for more oppression—not for ending the sexual and reproductive subordination of women.

When pornography and surrogacy are idealized as choices, this defines a new range of conformity for women. Choice is not the same as self-determination. Choice can be conformity if women have little ability to determine the conditions of consent. A woman may consent to use the pill or the IUD [intrauterine device] as a contraceptive, after having the risks explained to her, but she has no sexual and reproductive self-determination if she cannot say no to intercourse with her male partner. A woman who signs a surrogate contract, agreeing to bear a child for a contracting couple, consents to the arrangement, but she has little self-determination if she cannot find sustaining and dignified work and resorts to surrogacy as a final economic resort. Feminists must go beyond choice and consent as a standard for women's freedom. Before consent, there must be self-determination so that consent does not simply amount to acquiescing to the available options.

When technological reproduction perpetuates the role of women as breeders or encourages women to have children at any cost, this is not reproductive self-determination. It is conformity to old social roles garbed in new technologies and the new language of individual rights and choice. Under the guise of fostering procreative liberty, these reproductive arrangements help mold women to traditional reproductive roles. The fact that this compliance is ratified with the victim's consent only serves to emphasize how deeply conformity is entrenched and concealed in a gender-defined society.

Technological and contractual reproduction promotes the ideology that the problem of infertility *cannot* be confronted on an autonomous level but needs the intervention of medical and technical specialists to remedy the lack of biological children. Other options—an existence without children, an informed adoption—are not promoted as favorable alternatives. And thus women are left with the hollow rhetoric of choice—in reality, no choice at all.

Chapter 4

Do Reproductive Technologies Result in the Unethical Treatment of Embryos?

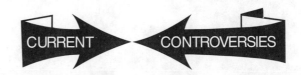

Genetic Screening of Embryos: An Overview

by Anita Cecchin

About the author: *Anita Cecchin is a writer for* Medical World News, *a health care periodical published in New York City.*

In the late 1970s, Americans grappled with the science and ethics of the first test-tube babies—babies born from embryos produced by in vitro fertilization. The goal of IVF then: to help parents with fertility problems have children.

Americans now face a new set of ethical questions as the next generation of test-tube babies—embryo-tested IVF babies—are born. The goal now: to produce babies free of their parents' genetic disorders.

At first glance, both goals have noble intentions, says Arthur Caplan, Ph.D., director of biomedical ethics at the University of Minnesota, Minn. "But as genetic testing of embryos improves and the Human Genome Project marches along, parents are going to ask, 'hey, what about picking traits that we consider desirable?' And is medicine going to get involved with that kind of goal?"

The new technique for screening embryos for genetic disorders prior to their implantation in the uterus will also fuel the abortion debate, says Baruch Brody, Ph.D., director of the Center for Ethics, Medicine, and Public Issues at Baylor College of Medicine in Houston.

"I think that first and foremost, the people participating in the abortion debate will be most interested in this new technique."

With this new technique, called preimplantation genetic diagnosis, parents who are at risk for certain inheritable disorders, such as cystic fibrosis or the X-linked disorders of hemophilia and Lesch-Nyhan syndrome, avoid transmitting them to their fetuses.

First, embryos, developed through regular IVF methods, are biopsied and then genetically analyzed by polymerase chain reaction testing. Then, unaffected embryos are implanted into the uterus so that the fetus is free of the parents' genetic disorder.

Anita Cecchin, "IVF Babies—the Next Generation," *Medical World News*, November 1992. Reprinted with permission of Miller Freeman Publishing, San Francisco.

In September 1992, doctors at London's Hammersmith Hospital and Baylor College of Medicine in Houston reported in the *New England Journal of Medicine* that a couple in England who were carriers for cystic fibrosis and who had their preimplanted embryos screened for that disorder had given birth in March 1992 to a normal baby girl.

And in October 1992, doctors at the Cornell University Medical College in New York announced the birth in August 1992 of the first baby in America to benefit from embryonic screening. The baby, a healthy 9 lb 3 oz girl, was born to a carrier of hemophilia who participated in an embryonic screening trial at Cornell.

Concerns About Selective Breeding

Despite the politically charged debate surrounding the abortion issue, embryonic screening should not have onerous implications, at least not in England, according to Alan Handyside, Ph.D., a senior lecturer at the Institute of Obstetrics and Gynaecology of Hammersmith Hospital in London.

In 1990, the British Parliament passed a law banning such research if the sole goal was merely to "enhance future generations," the same year Dr. Handyside first began screening embryos carried by women whose offspring could be at risk for X-linked recessive disorders. Only unaffected female embryos were implanted.

> *"Embryonic screening should not have onerous implications."*

But concerns that embryonic screening will lead to selective breeding or "genetic cleaning" still exist in the United States, Dr. Handyside said. "It's still a dilemma for Americans because your government has not passed a similar law."

Nonetheless, Dr. Mark Hughes of Baylor said embryonic screening offers a new alternative to Americans who may face legislation that is too restrictive on abortion or who do not want to consider aborting a fetus that has a genetic disorder.

"Their options before were limited," said Dr. Hughes, who heads the prenatal genetics program at Baylor and its affiliated Methodist Hospital in Houston. "First, they could adopt. Second, in the case of autosomal recessive disorders, they could use artificial insemination with an anonymous donor who did not carry the disease. Third, they could just throw the genetic dice and take a chance."

Dr. Hughes argues that the rights of parents to use embryonic screening should not be hampered by ethical questions. "I think of this research as being on the continuum of prenatal diagnosis," he said. "We've gone from amniocentesis (performed after 15 weeks' gestation) to chorionic-villus sampling (performed during the first trimester) to a test now that can be done before a clinical pregnancy. It's always been the objective to make the diagnosis earlier and earlier in pregnancy, even before a pregnancy, if possible."

That factor makes embryonic screening an ideal alternative for parents who oppose abortion, according to Dr. Michael Policar, vice president for medical affairs of the Planned Parenthood Federation of America. "The majority of people in this country feel that a fetus actually becomes a person somewhat later than the embryonic stage," he said. "I think without a doubt that there are many people who would not object to disposing of a 4- to 8-cell embryo when in fact they would have that problem later in the pregnancy."

Comparing Costs

However, surgeon Dr. Mildred Jefferson, a founding member of the Right-to-Life anti-abortion movement and a 1992 Republican congressional candidate from California, said that the development of embryonic screening may encourage insurance companies or the government to force parents with genetic disorders to have an embryonic test before pregnancy. She also expressed concern that only pregnancies from unaffected embryos would be insured in order to avoid the high costs of raising an ill child. "If you make it possible, that will be the mind-set of certain bureaucrats," Dr. Jefferson said.

According to a 1992 survey commissioned by Congress from the Office of Technology Assessment, the annual costs of caring for a child with mild to severe cystic fibrosis range from $8,500 to $46,000. That compared with a one-time $6,000 to $13,000 price tag for embryonic screening per IVF cycle.

"There's no doubt that embryo testing is a cost saver," Dr. Caplan said.

But cost savings should not be the driving force for future research, argues Robert Bell, Ph.D., of the Cystic Fibrosis Foundation. "In fact, this preimplantation technology is not an issue for us," he said. "Instead, we're focusing on new therapy for those 30,000 Americans already born with cystic fibrosis. The research we support offers so much hope not only for the current patient population but for affected individuals born in the future." Dr. Bell said 8 million Americans are carriers of the cystic fibrosis gene and that 1,000 babies with the disorder are born each year.

Although the price tag on preimplantation genetic diagnosis pales in comparison to the lifelong costs of caring for a CF sufferer, the procedure is still prohibitively expensive for most people. "We've been able to perform embryonic testing since March 1992 and more than 100 couples have asked about it. But we haven't had a single patient who could manage the cost," said Dr. Susan Black, clinical director of genetic preimplantation at the Genetics

> *"Concerns that embryonic screening will lead to selective breeding . . . still exist."*

& IVF Institute in Fairfax, Va. She said this is a contentious issue that continues to compromise their marketing efforts.

In England, the costs for embryonic screening are paid in part by private hospital trust funds and by the government's National Health Service. But in the

United States, Dr. Black said, Americans have to pay the total costs themselves. "For parents who know they're carriers because they already have an affected child, the cost can be something that is too hard to handle," she said.

Dr. Black insists that insurers so far have ignored evidence that embryonic screening may be less costly than funding the lifelong care of a severely ill patient.

Donald White, a spokesman for the Health Insurers Association of America, a trade association of commercial health insurers, says that it is not the savings that insurers are disputing, but rather the experimental nature of embryonic screening.

Said White, "We would probably cover it if it became standard medical practice. We're as far from that point as possible. It's not a matter of cost savings, or information, or education. It's a case of not dealing with standard medical practice."

Baylor's Dr. Hughes agrees that his research is cutting-edge medicine. "This is certainly still in the research stages. It's not the kind of situation where we're encouraging people to call an 800 number for more information," he said.

Allowing Parents to Genetically Screen Embryos Is Unethical

by Vicki G. Norton

About the author: *Vicki G. Norton, a 1994 graduate of the University of California–Los Angeles School of Law, is an attorney in La Jolla, California. She has a doctorate in biochemistry.*

> *Between the conception*
> *And the creation . . .*
> *Between the potency*
> *And the existence*
> *Between the essence*
> *And the descent*
> *Falls the Shadow.*
> —T.S. Eliot (1936)

Innovative reproductive technology has allowed Michelle and Paul O'Brien of Burnley, England to become the first parents to select their "test-tube" baby's genetic makeup. The recently developed technology—preimplantation genetic screening ("PGS")—combines *in vitro* fertilization ("IVF") techniques with genetic screening techniques to enable parents to predetermine their child's genetic traits. Without this technology, the O'Briens would have had a one in four chance of having a child with cystic fibrosis, but by using genetic screening, the O'Briens were able to select a disease-free embryo from among other embryos fertilized in a test-tube. Doctors then implanted the disease-free embryo into Michelle O'Brien, who gave birth to a healthy baby, named Chloe, in March of 1992. Although Chloe's parents used the technique for therapeutic purposes, the availability of such technology has raised concerns about its use for eugenic purposes, such as selecting a child's eye or hair color, or intelligence.

One other factor contributing to concern over the possible use of PGS as a eugenic tool is the progress of the three billion dollar government-funded Human

Excerpted from "Unnatural Selection: Nontherapeutic Preimplantation Genetic Screening and Proposed Regulation" by Vicki G. Norton, *UCLA Law Review*, vol. 41, no. 6, 1994. Reprinted with permission.

Genome Project. It is likely that the Human Genome Project will ultimately lead to the identification of the 50,000 to 100,000 genes found in the human genome. It could also facilitate parents' use of preimplantation screening to select a child's nontherapeutic genetic traits. As scientists sequence the human genome, they can identify and develop markers for those genes that are involved in genetic diseases. At the same time, scientists can also begin to identify and to develop markers for genes that determine cosmetic traits such as eye color, and for genes that play a role in "performance" traits, such as intelligence or artistic talent.

Even those in charge of the Human Genome Project have recognized the dangers inherent in genetic information. During her tenure as the Director of the National Institutes of Health ("NIH"), Dr. Bernadine Healy remarked, "Like fire . . . all powerful tools can be dangerous if misused or abused, and biomedicine's new molecular tools are no exception." As a result of these concerns, the NIH has set up a program of Ethical, Legal and Social Implications ("ELSI") as part of the National Center for Human Genome Research. The ELSI will assess the ethical and social implications of genetic identification techniques. The Genome Center has already recognized the need to prevent discrimination based on genetic makeup, and that such discrimination "is ethically no different from discrimination based on other biological traits such as gender, skin color, or disability."

A Lack of Regulation

While Congress has considered regulating genetic information or reproductive technology in other contexts, legislators have not yet proposed legislation to regulate the use of PGS for nontherapeutic purposes—that is, for purposes other than to insure the absence of genetic disease. For instance, the potential for the misuse of genetic information by employers or insurance companies has led Congress to consider passing the Human Genome Privacy Act. That Act would safeguard against the unauthorized use of genetic records maintained by government agencies, and would also insure that an individual has access to government agency records kept on that individual. In addition, the House of Representatives Committee on Government Operations has heard testimony on whether the Americans with Disabilities Act would prevent employer discrimination based on genetic makeup. However, neither the

> *"Even those in charge of the Human Genome Project have recognized the dangers inherent in genetic information."*

Human Genome Privacy Act nor the Americans with Disabilities Act would regulate PGS. Furthermore, in the Fertility Clinic Success Rate and Certification Act of 1992, which regulates *in vitro* fertilization clinics, Congress also failed to explicitly address the potential problems of preimplantation screening.

State legislatures have similarly focused their attention primarily on the prevention of the discriminatory use of genetic information by employers or insurance companies. While half of the states have passed laws prohibiting experimentation on fetuses or embryos, few, if any, of those laws would prevent the misuse of PGS of embryos. For example, the Utah legislature has specifically regulated the use of genetic screening of fetuses by prohibiting experimentation on "live unborn children," except to administer genetic tests required for therapeutic reasons. However, it is likely that the term "live unborn children" does not apply to early embryos that have not yet been implanted. Most of the other state statutes prohibiting fetal experimentation only prohibit experimentation on aborted fetuses or "live" unborn children and could not be used to regulate genetic screening of the preimplantation embryo. Yet the dangers inherent in PGS should not be ignored.

The History of Genetic Discrimination

The "eugenics movement" early in the twentieth century stands as a monument to the misuse of genetic information, when the fledgling field of genetics provided "evidence" for those seeking "proof" of the inferiority of unpopular minorities. A 1926 display by the American Eugenics Society contained a board on which a light flashed every fifteen seconds. The Society intended each flash of light to represent $100 of observers' money spent on caring for the "genetically inferior"—the Society wanted to encourage states to sterilize the genetically inferior to

> *"Congress . . . failed to explicitly address the potential problems of preimplantation screening."*

improve the gene pool, and to save the government the cost of caring for the inferior offspring of such individuals. Eventually the eugenics movement led to the passage of laws providing for the mandatory sterilization of "genetically inferior" criminals and the feeble-minded, prohibitions on interracial marriages, and the passage of the Immigration Restriction Act by Congress to restrict the immigration of "genetically inferior" individuals of non-Anglo-Saxon European descent.

Even the Supreme Court demonstrated an intolerance for genetically "inferior" individuals. In a 1927 case, Buck v. Bell, the Court upheld a Virginia law calling for sterilization of institutionalized inmates afflicted with a hereditary form of insanity or imbecility. In the opinion which rejected Carrie Buck's claim that such mandatory sterilization was unconstitutional, Justice Oliver Wendell Holmes wrote: "Three generations of imbeciles are enough."

Discrimination based on genetic makeup has persisted. The nation's treatment of carriers for sickle cell anemia is another stark example of the abuse of genetic information. In the 1970's, African Americans who were carriers for sickle cell anemia suffered discrimination which included denial of admission into the Air Force Academy, relegation to ground jobs by major airlines, and increased insurance costs. Individuals who carry other genetic diseases have also suffered discrimination. One couple who would have had a one in four chance of having a child with cystic fibrosis requested that their insurer pay for genetic testing of their fetus. The insurer agreed to pay only on the condition that the woman abort the fetus if it tested positive for the disease.

"The dangers inherent in PGS [preimplantation genetic screening] should not be ignored."

In light of the history of the excesses of eugenic programs and discrimination based on genetic makeup, there is a need to pass legislation which would prevent abuses of genetic screening. In particular, this article explores the need to regulate nontherapeutic PGS, with its potential for furthering discriminatory practices and eugenic goals. . . .

Moral Objections to Nontherapeutic PGS

Many of the moral arguments against the use of prenatal diagnosis and nontherapeutic selective abortion are equally applicable to the use of nontherapeutic PGS. Both procedures involve the use of sophisticated medical technology to assist parents in making a decision of life or death for the embryo based on factors unrelated to the health of the mother or the potential child. Also, in both procedures there would be no medical indication to perform the "diagnosis" and parents would be making their selection on the basis of factors other than a genetic risk to the fetus. In addition, there would be no potential harm to the family in the traditional sense of imposing the burden of caring for a sick child. This section discusses those moral objections which are equally applicable to selective abortions and nontherapeutic PGS because of these shared characteristics.

Scientists, ethicists, and the President's Commission for the Study of Ethical Problems in Medicine and Biomedical and Behavioral Research have advised against using fetal diagnosis for sex selection because it offends notions of gender equality. More generally, ethicists have advocated regulating selective abortions to protect against discrimination and to avoid its use for eugenic purposes. In addition, prenatal diagnosis and selective abortion may lead to parents viewing children as a means to an end, rather than as children to be accepted unconditionally. In fact, one set of doctors who were asked to carry out prenatal diagnosis for tissue matching concluded that "prenatal diagnosis should not be used to benefit a third party or facilitate the conception or abortion of a fetus for the purpose of generating an organ for transplantation."

One can raise similar moral objections to the use of nontherapeutic PGS. For instance, the use of preimplantation diagnosis for nontherapeutic purposes including sex selection may also lead to "discrimination" based on gender and other genetically determined traits. The ability to select traits in children raises

118

questions and fears about the motivations of those empowered to make such choices. When taken to an extreme, selection based on genetic makeup has led to atrocities such as the eugenic program carried out by Nazi Germany, in which it killed millions and sterilized hundreds of thousands in an attempt to get rid of "undesirables" of Jewish descent. The private use of nontherapeutic PGS would not lead to genocide; nevertheless, it does contain the potential for abuse as parents substitute their choice for natural selection. A form of "racial" discrimination would even be possible, if parents began selecting for cosmetic traits such as skin color or bone structure, which have traditionally been used to "identify" racial makeup. Regulation of nontherapeutic PGS would prevent parents from choosing between embryos on the basis of these or other genetic traits which are unrelated to disease.

Another moral objection which applies to PGS is that the technology may result in children becoming a means to achieve their parents' goals. If access to PGS were unrestricted, parents could choose traits in their children, much as animal breeders have "unconsciously" selected traits in animals for humankind's use. By selecting animals for breeding on the basis of phenotype, humankind has altered the characteristics of animals such as the thoroughbred horse. Humankind now has the ability to take "unconscious" selection a step further to "unnatural" selection by directly choosing the genetic makeup which will give rise to the desired characteristics.

> *"There is a need to pass legislation which would prevent abuses of genetic screening."*

However, animals bred by humankind have been bred for humankind's *use*. It is troubling to think that parents will begin selecting traits in children for either the parents' aesthetic "use" or for financial gain. Although parents have children for many reasons, there is a fine line between wanting a child to be the "best he can be" and wanting to bear a talented child whose talents can be financially exploited. It would be analogous to slavery if parents began selecting children on the basis of their earning potential in order to exploit it. Alternatively, it is possible that parents who select a talented child may care for their child as well as or better than parents who do not select their children, since the parents will have greater appreciation for the child's talents. Also, not all parents who select performance traits in a child will select those traits solely because they increase the child's earning potential. Nevertheless, the parents' unconditional love of a child is preferable to the parents' use of the child to satisfy the parents' personal desires. . . .

Banning Nontherapeutic Genetic Screening

Progress on the Human Genome Project will facilitate the development of new genetic markers for use in genetic screening, as well as help scientists to unravel the mechanisms of genetic diseases. Genetic screening is a powerful tool; its potential for aiding the search for cures for genetic diseases makes it invaluable. But we must not blindly embrace this technology. Rather, its potential uses must be harmonized with the interests of the government in genetic diversity, potential lives, and equal treatment for potential lives.

In light of the potential for the misuse of nontherapeutic PGS, and the absence of applicable statutes, Congress and state legislatures should take steps to ban nontherapeutic PGS. Such legislation should carefully define the term "nontherapeutic" to avoid its application to diagnostic procedures which are beneficial to the mother or child and to avoid unconstitutional vagueness. . . .

> *"Congress and state legislatures should take steps to ban nontherapeutic PGS."*

In speaking of the strides in technology which will be made by scientists participating in the Human Genome Project, George G. Gekas cautioned the House of Representatives that:

> The Human Genome Project will provide us with almost unimaginable opportunities to learn things about our DNA. Along with that new information comes new responsibilities. . . . Are we striving for the perfect human being? No! And will we become a society that will tolerate no less? I hope not. We do know that in both biology and society, difference is the rule rather than the exception. . . . By exploring the molecular details of the human race, we will not only marvel at our uncanny similarities but also celebrate our remarkable diversity.

As our society struggles with the implications of discoveries that expand the boundaries of science and the law, we should not lose sight of the abuses that can occur when intolerance becomes the rule. If we remember to "celebrate our remarkable diversity," and to strive for excellence rather than perfection, then we can responsibly explore the mysteries of our DNA, and put our scientific knowledge to valuable use.

Genetic Screening of Embryos Could Harm Society

by Regina Kenen

About the author: *Regina Kenen is a professor of sociology at Trenton State College in Trenton, N.J. She serves as liaison between the Council for Responsible Genetics and the National Women's Health Network.*

We live in the age of the Technological Imperative where existence of genetic diagnostic or screening tests seems to automatically translate into the expansion of these services for pregnant women. Although genetic services are presented as furthering women's choices the pressures to use these tests may actually constrain their ability to choose. The new technologies are increasingly influencing reproductive decision-making in the United States and pose ethical questions for women/couples who are planning to have a child.

Maps

Concern about the overuse or misuse of reproductive genetic technology is widespread and has escalated in recent years as a result of the Human Genome Project (HGP), a 15-year, $3-billion research effort to map and sequence the estimated 50,000 to 100,000 genes that make up the human genome. The goal of the HGP is to locate all the genes in the hope of determining their functions. To do this, scientists need to construct two types of maps—genetic linkage and physical maps.

Genetic linkage maps show how frequently individual diseases and other traits are inherited together within families over several generations. Advances in molecular genetics allow scientists to use "markers" (unique segments of DNA) that can be followed in families as landmarks on a genetic map. If they lie close to the yet unidentified gene suspected of causing the disease, they are likely to be inherited together.

Regina Kenen, "The Genetic Reproductive Technology Scene," (slightly revised by author) *Network News*, September/October 1993; © 1993 by the National Women's Health Network. Reprinted by permission.

Physical maps give the actual distances between genes on a chromosome. It is not enough to know where the genes are located; it is also necessary to understand their precise functioning. Determining the order of the nucleotides in a gene's DNA is known as sequencing, and this order determines the genetic information the gene carries.

Although the HGP focuses mainly on mapping and sequencing genes, it is the application of this knowledge that invokes apprehension. In fact, Congress was so concerned about the social use of the information arising out of the Human Genome Project that for the first time in history, it included a provision mandating that at least 3% of the money appropriated each year for the scientific project be spent on social, ethical and legal implications.

In addition, nationally known scientists, physicians, social scientists and women's health activists troubled by the possible social implications of genetic tests formed the Council for Responsible Genetics in 1983. The Council's purpose is to alert the public to the social issues raised by genetic technology and to promote discussion about these issues, many of which impact women. Two primary areas of concern are the overuse of genetic tests in the clinical setting and the erroneous interpretations and misuse of the test information by third parties.

The Carrier Label

As we all know, we inherit our genes from our biological parents and hand them down to our biological children. Some genetic diseases are carried on a dominant gene. This means that a child only has to inherit that gene from one parent in order to have the specific condition. Other diseases, such as Tay-Sachs or cystic fibrosis, are carried on recessive genes, which means the harmful gene must be inherited from both parents in order for a child to develop the disease. In that case, if a child only inherits one gene, then he or she is a carrier of that disease, a person who can pass the gene on to another generation, but who will never actually develop the condition himself or herself. Geneticists estimate that each one of us carries four to eight recessive genes that could cause conditions detrimental to our health. That makes it likely that as more genetic tests come on the market, all of us will be at risk of becoming identified as carriers of genetic conditions.

> *"The new [reproductive] technologies . . . pose ethical questions for women/couples who are planning to have a child."*

Most of us know that individuals with a genetic condition or disability experience discrimination in their everyday lives. Yet, few of us are aware that "carriers" of genetic conditions also experience discrimination. Sometimes people who are just at risk of being a carrier for a severe genetic disease are discriminated against if a member of the family is known to be affected. One woman had an uncle who had been diagnosed recently as having Huntington's disease (a dominant genetic defect which expresses itself in mid-life and leads to physical and mental deterioration and death), and was seeking medical information for her mother. She lost her own medical insurance and was unable to obtain life insurance when her insurance company found out about her uncle's condition. This story gives us a glimpse into how vulnerable we are to invasion of our privacy by interested third parties.

Genes and the Environment

To complicate matters further, most diseases involve both genetic and environmental factors. Even though we constantly read and hear about how genetic discoveries will provide firm answers, the reality is different. Answers will not be clear cut. Human beings are not Mendelian peas. Cultural, social and environmental influences interact with genes, and genes interact with the rest of the cell. Thus, scientific and medical predictions of the future for individuals with certain genetic conditions may not be accurate. When large numbers of individuals are genetically diagnosed as being "at high risk" of developing specific diseases, but with no certainty that they will ever develop them, the stage is set for stigmatization and discrimination.

> *"Human beings are not Mendelian peas."*

Despite academic discussions about how diverse people with the same genetic condition can be, a genetic diagnostic test is usually interpreted in terms of the worst possible outcome. For example, most people think of a child with cystic fibrosis (an inherited, chronic disease of the pancreas and the lungs) as being sick most of the time and dying before the age of thirty. Although this is true for many, the outlook is much better for others. It was this worst case scenario that obsessed one health maintenance organization (HMO). The HMO was not very pleased when a patient decided not to abort her fetus when it tested positive for cystic fibrosis. Instead of offering her additional information about the disease and support services, the HMO informed her that her decision would limit her coverage for the pregnancy, and care of the new baby, and possibly even future care for herself, her husband and previous child. So much for our just and caring health care system!

Particular controversy surrounds genetic testing for diseases when environmental influences as well as genetic predispositions appear to play a role, such as in some forms of breast cancer. Rather than concentrating on the role of genes in breast cancer, many women's health activists believe that more emphasis should be placed on identifying cultural, social and environmental factors that might also play a role. A new study published in the *Journal of the American Medical Association* affirms that position. The findings indicate that even when there is a family history of breast cancer, environment can still play a large role in interacting with the genetic makeup.

Social decisions as well as scientific ones determine the areas on which we focus our scientific resources. Currently, we are riding a genetic bandwagon that overemphasizes the genetic components of health problems to the detriment of other areas of inquiry.

Addressing Women's Needs

New technologies must address women's needs. If used appropriately, they can be beneficial to many. Diagnostic tests can also cause anxiety, provoke conflicts among family members and raise questions about the importance of the "perfect" biological child. In many cases it is society's attitude toward people with "disabilities" more than the "disability" itself that becomes the major handicap.

The number of genes responsible for genetic diseases that can be detected by screening tests and prenatal diagnosis in carriers continues to grow. In addition, the definition of what is considered a genetic flaw expands along with technological progress. This means that what previously may have been seen as a "difference" is now labeled a "defect." Improvements in effectively treating or preventing many disorders are increasing, although at a slower pace. Some scientists believe that for certain genetic conditions, there may be as long as a 50-year lag between carrier detection and prenatal diagnosis and a cure.

Yet, industry analysts estimate that over the next 10 years, as many as 18 million individuals will be screened for carrier status, chromosome abnormalities and common genetic predispositions (e.g., insulin-dependent diabetes, breast cancer). As people buy into the idea that genes are the most important cause of disease and disability, less energy, money and motivation will be spent seeking answers in the cultural, social and environmental realms, and prevention will mean prevention of the birth of those considered genetically inferior. As reproductive issues are at stake, the pressure to use the new technology and the burden of decision-making will rest primarily on women.

Experimenting on Embryos Is Unethical

by The Ramsey Colloquium

About the author: *The Ramsey Colloquium is a group of Jewish and Christian theologians, philosophers, and scholars who meet periodically to consider questions of ethics, religion, and public life. The colloquium is sponsored by the Institute on Religion and Public Life.*

A panel of nineteen experts appointed by the National Institutes of Health has recommended government funding for conceiving human embryos in the laboratory for the sole purpose of using them as materials for research. After carefully studying the Report of the Human Embryo Research Panel, we conclude that this recommendation is morally repugnant, entails grave injustice to innocent human beings, and constitutes an assault upon the foundational ideas of human dignity and rights essential to a free and decent society. The arguments offered by the Panel are more ideological and self-interested than scientific; the actions recommended by the Panel cross the threshold into a world of apparently limitless technological manipulation and manufacture of human life. The Panel claims to draw a "clear line" against experiments that almost everyone would deem abhorrent. In fact it does not draw such a line and, by virtue of its own logic, it cannot draw such a line. The recommendation, if adopted, will be a fateful step for humanity from which it may be impossible to turn back.

All of us have a stake in the questions raised. In a society such as ours, these questions cannot be, they must not be, decided by a committee of experts. We urge a comprehensive public debate and intense congressional scrutiny regarding the proposals emanating from the NIH. The research recommended by the Panel should not be funded by the government. It should not be done at all. It should be prohibited by law. In what follows we attempt to explain how we have reached this conclusion.

We are confident that most people, to the extent that they are aware of the Panel's recommendation, experience an immediate and strong revulsion. This is

Excerpted and reprinted with permission from "The Inhuman Use of Human Beings" by the Ramsey Colloquium, which originally appeared in the January 1995 issue of *First Things*, a monthly journal published by the Institute on Religion and Public Life, New York, N.Y.

not to be dismissed as an irrational reaction. It signals a deep, intuitive awareness of lines that must not be crossed if we are to maintain our sometimes frag-
ile hold upon our own humanity.

For instance, the *Washington Post*'s editorial response to the Panel's proposal
declared flatly that "The creation of human embryos specifically for research
that will destroy them is unconscionable." The acids of moral relativism have
not advanced so far in our culture as to destroy completely the capacity to know
and say that *some things are simply not to be countenanced*, much less approved and funded by the government. The editorial goes on to distinguish the
present question from that of abortion. "To suggest that support for abortion
rights equals support for such [embryo] experimentation is to buy abortion opponents' view that permitting abortion means erasing society's ability to make
distinctions." The question of creating, using, and destroying human embryos
cannot be separated entirely from the question of abortion, but the two questions can and should be distinguished. We hope that most people, whatever
their views on the legalization of abortion, will be moved to take a stand at this
new line that must not be crossed.

The ominously new thing in the Panel's Report is that embryonic human life
should be treated simply as research material to be used and discarded—and
should even be brought into being solely for that purpose. The Report readily
acknowledges that the embryos to be used are instances of human life. It does
not hesitate to answer the question of when a new human life begins. Indeed,
indisputable scientific evidence leaves no choice: a new human life begins at
conception (or, as the Report usually prefers, "fertilization"). The Report
speaks of the embryo from the earliest moment as "developing human life." We
are at various points told that the very early embryo deserves "serious moral
consideration," "moral respect," "profound respect," and "some added measure
of respect beyond that accorded animal subjects."

The Embryo Is Human

Honesty requires that we speak not simply of human life but of a human being. Skin and intestinal tissue, even eggs and sperm, are human life. But, unlike
such instances of human life, the embryo from the earliest moment has the active capacity to articulate itself into
what everyone acknowledges is a human being. The embryo is a being;
that is to say, it is an integral whole
with actual existence. The being is
human; it will not articulate itself

> *"Human beings are always to be treated as ends and never merely as means."*

into some other kind of animal. Any being that is human is a human being. If it
is objected that, at five days or fifteen days, the embryo does not look like a human being, it must be pointed out that this is precisely what a human being
looks like—and what each of us looked like—at five or fifteen days of develop-

ment. Clarity of language is essential to clarity of thought.

The question is whether the government should permit and fund the production of human beings—completely innocent and powerless human beings—to be used as material for scientific research. After answering that question in the affirmative, the Report then considers which human beings can be so used and which cannot. It is one of the most treasured maxims of our civilization that human beings are al-

> *"Every human being is inviolable."*

ways to be treated as ends and never merely as means. In a partial dissent from the Report, Professor Patricia A. King, a member of the Panel, writes, "The fertilization of human oocytes [female eggs] for research purposes is unnerving because human life is being created solely for human *use*. I do not believe that this society has developed the conceptual frameworks necessary to guide us down this slope. . . . At the very least, we should proceed with extreme caution." The conclusion that properly follows from her fully justified anxiety is that we should proceed not at all. Regrettably, the other members of the Panel appear not to have shared even the anxiety.

In weighing the question of which human beings can be used as a means to the ends of scientific progress and which cannot, the Report says the decision must rest on a "multi-factorial" judgment. By this is meant that no one principle or line of reasoning will support the conclusion that the Panel reaches. The Report's use of "multi-factorial" judgment is tantamount to suggesting that an accumulation of doubtful arguments will produce a convincing conclusion. In the course of reaching its "multi-factorial" judgment, the Panel entangles itself in philosophical, moral, and even scientific confusions. We are sorry to report that, in some of its arguments, the Panel invites the charge of being more than a little disingenuous.

"Personhood"

In order to decide which human embryos are usable and which are "protectable" from such use, the Report leans very heavily on the concept of "personhood." The question is switched from "When does the life of a human being begin?" to "When does a human being become a person?" Persons are protectable; nonpersons or those who are deemed to be something less than persons are not protectable. But the only reason they are not protectable is that they will not be protected. Although they are obviously protectable in the sense that we are capable of protecting them, they are designated "not protectable" because we have decided not to protect them. And we decide not to protect them because they are not persons. Whether they are persons, and therefore protectable, depends upon their possessing certain qualities that we associate with persons and think worth protecting. Here and elsewhere in the Report, the reader is struck by a large measure of circularity in the Panel's reasoning.

The question is not whether the embryo is protectable but whether it is in need of protection. The Report says that "the commencement of protectability is not an all or nothing matter, but results from a being's increasing possession of qualities that make respecting it (and hence limiting others' liberty in relation to it) more compelling." In other words, moral standing develops as the human being develops, and "personhood" is an award we bestow for performance. The principle espoused by the Report leads to the suggestion that our obligation to afford protection to a human being is in inverse proportion to his or her need for protection. Put differently, those who are fully and undoubtedly persons are protectable because they are, by and large, able to protect themselves.

It is not traditional in ethical discourse to discuss what "life" or "forms of life" or "developing forms of life" are entitled to respect and protection. Living human beings are so entitled. The classical conviction of our culture has been that, contrary to the Report, it is "an all or nothing matter." We are implicated in the fate of all; every human being is inviolable. It has taken society much blood and struggle to overcome what Professor King calls the "conceptual frameworks" whereby the powerful justified excluding various categories of the powerless from moral parity. The Panel's use of "personhood" is such a conceptual framework, and it applies to both the born and unborn.

The concept of personhood has a complicated history in theology, philosophy, and law. Personhood is certainly not a scientific concept. As used by the Panel, it is an ideological concept, an idea in the service of a program aimed at changing dramatically our civilization's understanding of human life and community. In this Report, personhood is a status that we bestow. We who have received that status decide who will be admitted to, and who will be excluded from, the circle of those who are recognized as persons and are therefore entitled to respect and protection. We are told that protectability increases with an "increasing possession of qualities" that we find compelling. It follows that protectability decreases with the decreasing possession of such qualities.

From their writings and public statements, we know that some members of the Panel do not flinch from the ominous implications of that principle for those who have lost their "compelling" qualities, especially at the end of the life spectrum. As a more complete explanation of its ethical reasoning, the Report cites an article by Professor Ronald Green, himself a member of the Panel, "Toward a Copernican Revolution in Our Thinking About Life's Beginning and Life's End." It is indeed a revolution that is proposed by Professor Green and by the Human Embryo Research Panel. The cited article asserts that there are no "qualities existing *out there*" in any human being requiring us to respect him or her as a person. Whether to grant or deny "personhood" (and hence the right not to be harmed or killed) is, we are told, "the outcome of a very active and complex

> *"What affects all should . . . be decided by all."*

process of decision on our part." In the current language of the academy, personhood is entirely a "social construct." Whether someone is too young or too old, too retarded or too sick, too troublesome or too useless to be entitled to personhood is determined by a "decision on our part." The American people have not been consulted about, and certainly have not consented to, this "Copernican Revolution" in our understanding of human dignity and human rights.

> *"The production of human beings for the purpose of experiments . . . should be prohibited by law."*

The revolution is necessary, however, in order to license, morally and legally, the research that the Panel recommends. The "conceptual frameworks" of the Report's extended ethical and philosophical reflection obscure rather than illumine the questions at hand. As already indicated, the question is not the difference between human beings who are persons and those who allegedly are not but the difference between human beings and other animals. Similarly, the Report makes much of the "preimplantation embryo" (implantation in the womb usually begins with the sixth day and is completed by the fourteenth day after conception). A "greater measure of respect" is due the embryo after the fourteenth day, says the Panel. This is gravely misleading. In question are not preimplantation embryos but *unimplanted* embryos—embryos produced with the intention that they will *not* be implanted and can therefore be kept alive and experimented upon as long as they are scientifically useful.

There are additional obfuscations. The Report makes much of the "twinning" factor. An early embryo is said not to be "individuated" because in a very small minority of cases the embryo may "twin" into two or more human beings. The ethical significance of this possibility is elusive. The fact that in rare instances an embryo may divide is no justification whatever for deliberately producing human embryos for the purpose of experimentation that will destroy them. Moreover, the Report repeatedly points to the "potential" of the embryo for further development as an indicator of whether or not it is "protectable." Here the circularity of reasoning is particularly blatant: A human being is not protectable in the early stages of development because, the Report claims, it has no potential for further development. But in the case of the embryo produced in the laboratory it has no potential for further development for the sole reason that researchers will not protect it. Because they wish to use it, they do not protect it; because they do not protect it, its natural potential for development is destroyed; because it thus "has no potential," it is declared "not protectable."

No Line Determines "Personhood"

The monumental questions raised by this Report—Who shall live and who shall die? Who belongs to the community of the commonly protected? How do we distinguish between human beings and laboratory animals?—demand much more serious thinking than is offered by the Human Embryo Research Panel.

The Panel claims to have established clear lines and clear time limits regarding what it is permissible to do with human embryos. That claim is false, and it seems that the panelists know that it is false. The Report says that research with these living human beings "should not be permitted beyond the time of the usual appearance of the primitive streak in vivo (14 days)." (The primitive streak is a groove that develops along the midline of the embryonic disc and its appearance is viewed as one of several milestones in the embryo's continuous development.) But this time limit is clearly arbitrary and chosen as a pragmatic compromise, as the transcript of the Panel's deliberations makes clear.

The panelists all know that development is continuous and it offers no such bright natural line to those who would "ascribe personhood." Moreover, this "time limit" is by no means firm, as is evident in the Report's assertion that it should serve "at the present time," and "for the foreseeable future." Some technically possible and scientifically interesting experiments "warrant additional review," while others are deemed "unacceptable for federal funding" because the desired experiments can at present be done with laboratory animals and because of "concern for public sensitivities on highly controversial research proposals." At the present time. For the foreseeable future.

> *"The proposal that some human beings should be declared 'not protectable' affects all of us."*

For example, producing genetically identical individuals to be born at different times, freezing an embryonic human being who is genetically identical to a born child in order to serve as a later source for organ and tissue transplantation, cloning an existing human being, and making "carbon copies" of an existing embryo—these and other projects are declared to be "inappropriate." It is not clear that the Report opposes the doing of these things; it simply does not recommend, at present, federal funding for doing them. But in the logic of the Report, there is no reason *in principle* why these things should not be done or why they should not be funded by the government.

"Throughout its deliberations," we are told, "the Panel relied on the principle that research involving preimplantation embryos is acceptable public policy only if the research promises significant scientific and therapeutic benefits." But a principle that says something should not be done unless there are strong motives for doing it is no principle at all. The claim to have set limits is vitiated by the repeated assertion that exceptions can be made for "serious and compelling reasons." The "Copernican Revolution" is nothing less than the abandonment of any and all principled limits. If it is for "serious and compelling reasons," scientists can do whatever they decide to do with human beings who are declared to be "unprotectable." And they can get government funding for doing it, within the limits of "public sensitivities." There is no reason, in principle, why such license would be confined to very small and very young human beings.

Of course the Panel believes that its recommendations are supported by "serious and compelling reasons" having to do with gains in scientific knowledge and therapeutic benefits. We do not doubt that lethal experiments on powerless and unconsenting human beings might result in findings of scientific interest. As for therapeutic benefits, the Report holds out the promise of improved success with in

> *"Concern for the interests of the subject must always prevail over the interest of science and society."*

vitro fertilization, new contraceptive techniques, new prospects for genetic screening, the production of cell lines for use in tissue transplantation, and, more vaguely, treatment of cancer and other diseases.

In fact, the Report seems too reticent in its discussion of possible "benefits" from the research it proposes. In a time when the entire human genome is being mapped, when the age is rising at which many women first become mothers, when, consequently, there is increased anxiety about the risk of genetic diseases, when harvesting parts from the embryo and fetus may have therapeutic uses for older human beings, when care for the handicapped and defective is viewed by many as excessively burdensome, and when it seems technically possible to produce custom-made babies—in such a time it is not surprising that people might be tempted to agree that the Panel's recommendations are supported by "serious and compelling reasons." The Report explicitly encourages funding for "preimplantation genetic screening," and the laboratory testing of artificially fertilized embryos before they are placed in the womb. The normalizing of in vitro fertilization and the universalizing of genetic screening in order to eliminate the unfit and advance eugenic goals are part of a "brave new world" clearly advanced by the proposals of the Human Embryo Research Panel. . . .

Our concern is with the philosophy and moral reasoning embraced by the Panel. Our conviction—and, we are confident, the conviction of almost all Americans—is that the ominous questions engaged must not be decided by one-sided committees of the National Institutes of Health. What affects all should, through our representative process, be decided by all. The proposal that some human beings should be declared "not protectable" affects all of us. The proposal that human beings should be treated merely as means rather than ends is revolutionary, but it is not new. Such "conceptual frameworks" have a terrifying history, not least in this bloodiest of centuries.

Research Should Be Banned

The production of human beings for the purpose of experiments that will destroy them should be prohibited by law. The use of human beings for experiments that will do them harm and to which they have not given their consent should be prohibited by law. It matters not how young or how small, how old or how powerless, such human beings may be. Some nations ban or severely restrict the research proposed by the Panel (e.g., Norway, Germany, Austria, Australia). In the shadow of the unspeakable horror of Nazism, the Nuremberg Code declared, "No experiment should be conducted where there is an a priori reason to believe that death or disabling injury will occur." And the 1975 Helsinki Declaration of the World Medical Association affirms, "Concern for the interests of the subject must always prevail over the interest of science and society."

It is objected that a ban would not be enforceable. If so, how can anyone believe that the proposed regulation by NIH would be enforceable? The research recommended by the Panel is now being done under various auspices, with or without government funding. Driven by scientific curiosity and hubris, reinforced by the prospect of great commercial gain and a belief that it will produce benefits for society, such research probably cannot be stopped altogether. But the necessity of a law does not depend on its being universally effective. What must be made illegal and declared morally odious is any research that subjects human beings to scientific experimentation that will certainly result in their grave injury or death.

The shamelessly partisan and conceptually confused Report of the Human Embryo Research Panel should be unambiguously rejected. Limits that are "for the present time" and "for the foreseeable future" limit nothing. They are but unconvincing reassurances that scientists are going carefully where they should not be permitted to go at all. If the course recommended by the Panel is approved, the foreseeable future is ominously clear: it is a return to the past when people contrived "conceptual frameworks" for excluding categories of human beings, born and unborn, from our common humanity.

Embryos Can Be Disposed of Ethically

by Jennifer P. Brown

About the author: *Jennifer P. Brown, a 1994 graduate of the University of San Francisco Law School, is an attorney in the Sacramento office of Orrick, Herrington, and Sutcliffe, a San Francisco law firm.*

The increasing use of in vitro fertilization ("IVF") as an alternative means of conception is creating a myriad of complex issues for the legal community. State legislatures, Congress and the courts have yet to adequately address questions raised by IVF technology. In particular, "cryopreservation," the practice of freezing preembryos fertilized during the IVF procedure for future implantation, is creating controversy.

During the IVF procedure, several eggs are retrieved from the woman's ovaries for subsequent fertilization and implantation. Although every egg retrieved is fertilized with donor sperm, to avoid multiple gestation, only three or four fertilized preembryos are immediately implanted in the woman's uterus. Cryopreservation permits the remaining fertilized preembryos to be preserved for future implantation if a successful pregnancy is not achieved with the initial IVF procedure.

The present debate involving cryopreservation and "frozen embryos" focuses on whether these preembryos may be discarded by gamete providers and whether mandatory donation of preembryos is constitutional. Thus far, only Louisiana and New Mexico have enacted legislation directly regulating the discard of cryopreserved embryos. By judicial decision or legislation several other jurisdictions have concluded that the destruction of preembryos is homicide or feticide by their definition of "fetus." A constitutional evaluation of such legislation necessarily involves difficult moral and ethical questions. . . .

Regulations prohibiting the discard of preembryos violate the biological donors' right to procreative liberty and, absent a compelling state interest, are unconstitutional. It is not the position of this article, however, that no regulation of IVF and cryopreservation should occur. The very nature of IVF and in particular, cryopreservation, demands that society take an active role in monitoring the IVF process to protect the integrity of the family structure and ensure that pregnancy and childrearing do not become wholly commercial ventures. Legislation requiring all fertilized preembryos to be implanted, however, infringes on the gamete providers' right to control their reproductive decisions and is therefore unconstitutional absent a compelling state interest and a narrowly drawn state statute. . . .

The Right to Avoid Procreation

The fundamental right to *avoid* procreation is central to the analysis of laws prohibiting preembryo discard because it is this right that gamete providers exercise when they choose not to implant a preembryo. Although the Supreme Court has not decided any cases directly addressing the gamete providers' right not to implant a preembryo, an examination of the Court's decisions recognizing a right to avoid pregnancy by way of contraception demonstrates the constitutional infirmity of state laws requiring mandatory donation and prohibiting the discard of preembryos.

The Court's recognition of a right to procreate in *Skinner* infers that if a person is not exercising a right *to* procreate, he or she is exercising a right *not* to procreate. The decision whether or not to procreate "is protected because of the importance of the biological and social experiences that bearing and rearing a child entails." Thus, state statutes that prohibit the destruction of preembryos violate the gamete providers' fundamental right to decide when and if they wish to become parents.

In *Davis v. Davis*, the Tennessee Court of Appeals and the Tennessee Supreme Court recognized that the right to procreate includes the right to avoid procreation. Both the court of appeals and the state supreme court based their conclusions in part on *Skinner v. Oklahoma*. Both courts reached the conclusion that there is a fundamental right to avoid procreation by examining the United States Supreme Court's decisions on reproductive rights.

The United States Supreme Court's rulings in *Griswold v. Connecticut* and *Eisenstadt v. Baird* established that an individual's decision whether to beget a child is fundamental to individual autonomy. The privacy interests involved in the decision not to implant a preembryo cannot be distinguished from privacy interests involved in the decision to use birth control.

> *"Regulations prohibiting the discard of preembryos . . . are unconstitutional."*

As the Court stated in *Eisenstadt*, the right to privacy "is the right of the *individual*, married or single, to be free from unwarranted governmental intrusion into matters so fundamentally affecting a person as the decision whether to bear or beget a child." Therefore, a state may not prohibit the destruction of a preembryo without violating the gamete providers' fundamental right to make reproductive decisions. The decision not to implant a preembryo is based on the same premise as the decision to use contraceptives: a desire not to bear or beget a child.

State statutes that provide for mandatory donation of preembryos if the gamete providers decide not to implant are in direct conflict with the United States Supreme Court's recognition in *Griswold* and *Eisenstadt* of a fundamental right to use contraception to refrain from bearing a child. The

> *"The right to procreate includes the right to avoid procreation."*

cryopreserved preembryo's stage of development at the time of freezing is similar to that of an embryo developing inside a woman's uterus prior to implantation in the uterine wall. Thus, if the Court has recognized a fundamental right to use contraceptives, some of which operate after fertilization, the decision not to implant the preembryo must be granted the same protections.

The Tennessee Supreme Court in *Davis v. Davis* relied on *Griswold* and *Eisenstadt* when it recognized a fundamental right to not procreate in the context of IVF. Using the Tennessee Constitution and federal case law as a foundation, the court held that inherent in the right to privacy is both the right to procreate and the right to avoid procreation. The court stated that the Supreme Court's "reproductive freedom" cases, such as *Griswold* and *Roe*, and the Court's decisions regarding parental rights and responsibilities with respect to children demonstrated "[t]hat a right to procreational autonomy is inherent in our most basic concepts of liberty. . . ."

No State Right to Control Procreation

The Supreme Court's holdings in the area of contraception, including *Eisenstadt*, *Griswold* and *Carey*, demonstrate the Court's commitment to the principle that a person has a fundamental right to make the decision to become a parent. The IVF process itself is the only difference between the privacy interests involved in the destruction of an IVF preembryo and the privacy interests recognized in the Court's contraception decisions. Just as no one, including a person's parents or marital partner, may preclude that person from using contraception to prevent pregnancy, the state may not affirmatively order cryopreserved embryos to be brought to life without depriving the individual seeking to avoid parental responsibility of the fundamental right to use a contraceptive.

The decision to discard a preembryo also cannot be distinguished from the decision to use a post-fertilization birth control device such the "morning-after pill." Although the Supreme Court has not directly addressed the constitutionality of post-fertilization birth control, access to other forms of contraception is a fundamental right under *Griswold* and its progeny. For the same reason that state statutes restricting the availability of contraceptives were invalidated by the Court, state statutes prohibiting the discard of preembryos and mandating adoptive implantation in the egg donor or a third party infringe on the fundamental right to control child-rearing decisions.

The fundamental right to avoid procreation encompasses the decision not to implant a preembryo. Mandatory donation laws and laws prohibiting the discard of preembryos infringe upon this right by stripping the gamete providers of their right to decide when and if they choose to become parents. The right to procreate necessarily encompasses the right to avoid procreation and the decision not to implant a preembryo is no different than the decision to use contraceptives. Because the United States Supreme Court has protected the right to procreate and the right to obtain contraceptives as fundamental, mandatory donation laws and laws prohibiting the discard of preembryos are unconstitutional. . . .

Left alone, cryopreserved embryos will never result in a live birth. An affirmative step must be taken to bring them to life. States may not assert a greater interest in protecting IVF preembryos than embryos fully implanted in a woman's uterus. Thus, increased recognition of the state interest in potential life does not affect the constitutionality of state laws prohibiting preembryo discard. Because the state interest in potential life does not constitute a compelling interest, state laws restricting preembryo discard cannot be upheld.

The State Cannot Force People to Become Parents

Mandatory donation laws and state regulations that act to prohibit the discard of preembryos confer more protection on preembryos than is justified under the Supreme Court's decisions recognizing a right to privacy in contraception and procreation. The gamete providers' authority to discard preembryos and thereby prevent their implantation is protected by the fundamental right not to procreate recognized in *Skinner v. Oklahoma*. This authority is also found in the contraceptive privacy cases because the preembryo is significantly less developed than, for example, the fertilized egg that is prevented from implantation in the uterus by an IUD. The Court's precedent that protects the right to bear a child coitally, logically includes the decision to bear a child by noncoital reproduction because the Court's recognition of this right protects not the coitus itself but the fundamental decision to bear a child.

> *"An individual's decision whether to beget a child is fundamental to individual autonomy."*

The Supreme Court recognized that the right to procreate includes the right to avoid procreation in its procreation, contraception and abortion decisions. There is little difference in terms of personal autonomy between the decision to prevent or terminate a pregnancy and the decision not to implant a preembryo. Both decisions emanate from a desire to avoid becoming a parent. Thus, the fundamental right to decide "whether to bear or beget a child" encompasses the decision not to implant a cryopreserved embryo.

Mandatory donation laws impose a substantial psychological burden on the gamete providers. State laws mandating adoptive implantation of preembryos or preventing their discard act in total disregard of the gamete providers' decision not to become parents. Even without the gestational and rearing responsibilities that normally accompany parenthood, gamete providers are forced to live with the fact that they have children—children with whom they will have no contact and no influence in their upbringing. While society has accepted this burden for persons who voluntarily surrender their parental rights under traditional adoption procedures, state mandated adoptive implantation of preembryos is both involuntary and a direct violation of the gamete providers' constitutional rights.

> *"Reproductive freedoms must be safeguarded from unwarranted state intervention and control."*

Reproductive freedoms must be safeguarded from unwarranted state intervention and control. As the success and utilization of alternative reproductive technologies increases, the debate over the legal status of the preembryo and the gamete providers' fundamental right to control the fate of their preembryos will continue. Laws prohibiting preembryo discard confer extraordinary power on the state. Such laws may prevent infertile couples from exercising their constitutionally protected right to become parents because gamete providers who are aware that their preembryos will be donated to strangers without their consent may forego alternative reproductive technologies altogether. The reproductive decisions of infertile couples must be granted the same constitutional protections as other couples if the benefits of alternative reproductive technologies are to be fully realized.

Allowing Parents to Genetically Screen Embryos Can Be Ethical

by Owen D. Jones

About the author: *Owen D. Jones is Associate Professor of Law at the Arizona State University School of Law.*

A line of Supreme Court cases culminating in *Planned Parenthood v. Casey* establishes that personal autonomy in reproductive matters is an important (though not absolute) social and legal value. *Casey* provides, in part, that the Constitution protects each person's autonomy in the realm of personal liberties vindicating the most basic decisions about "family," "parenthood," and "procreation."

Recent insights from evolutionary biology into the procedures and mechanisms by which humans reproduce, however, require an expanded understanding of what family parenthood, and procreation are all about. So long as the values articulated in *Casey* guide the incorporation of scientific observations into the legal analysis of laws directly affecting reproduction, evolutionary biology will profoundly affect the extent to which federal law protects an individual's access to reproductive technologies from government intrusion. Specifically, if the basis articulated in *Casey* for subjecting abortion laws to heightened judicial scrutiny is applied consistently, then the use of technologies to select specific traits in children should receive the same federal protection as that afforded abortion.

A number of provocative and process-oriented reproductive technologies, including fertility enhancement (by, for example, artificial insemination, surrogacy, or cryopreservation of embryos) and fertility control (by, for example, contraception, prevention of implantation, or abortion) have already inspired considerable debate in legal and ethical literature. Yet technology increasingly affords women (together, at times, with men) the power to influence the genetic makeup of children, and this presents novel questions with far-reaching impli-

From "Reproductive Autonomy and Evolutionary Biology: A Regulatory Framework for Trait-Selection Technologies" by Owen D. Jones, *American Journal of Law and Medicine*, vol. 19, no. 3, 1993. Excerpted and reprinted with permission of the American Society of Law, Medicine & Ethics and of the author.

cations for the social order.

The actual selection of offspring characteristics, using what might usefully be termed "trait-selection technologies" (TSTs), offers not merely the facilitation or prevention of birth, but rather its refinement. Sperm separation techniques, for example, are being used to skew the chances of having a male or female child. Genetic screening of embryos allows the abortion of fetuses with traits the parent finds undesirable. And gene splicing techniques and therapies appear to offer the promise that genes coded for characteristics a parent finds undesirable may soon be replaced with those coded for desired characteristics.

> *"The use of technologies to select specific traits in children should receive . . . federal protection."*

The foregoing technologies focus on the *product* (that is, the physical result), rather than on the *process*, of creation and reproduction. Ancient distinctions between reproduction and production are thus disappearing. Such a paradigm shift, from baby as indivisible package to baby as mix-and-match product, raises the specter of "designer" babies—and this pushes the limits of society's tolerance for diverse reproductive behavior.

Trait selection is neither simply speculative nor fully developed. TSTs are already used to influence the likelihood of a child manifesting certain traits. And the import and scope of TSTs are growing, fueled (in part) by the inexorable progress of ongoing efforts to map the entire human genome. Consequently, the proliferation of TSTs requires a careful inquiry to identify, understand, and evaluate the possible significance of the differences among them. . . .

If we generally value the liberty to make fundamental decisions about reproduction that are central to personal autonomy, as *Casey* indicates, then laws designed to prohibit or impede access to TSTs should be subject to heightened judicial scrutiny.

To see why this is so, one may consider a concrete, current, and controversial example in which certain TST is being used: sex selection. One must then explore several fundamental principles of evolutionary biology, which are relevant to any discussion of TST, and discuss how these affect our understanding and approach to sex selection, and illuminate TST issues in general.

A Current Example: Sex Selection

Sex selection in humans raises several themes that underlie any discussion of TSTs. It illuminates the ancient and powerful desire to control offspring and exemplifies the rapid, often awe-inspiring, pace of technology enabling trait selection. It also reveals the current and potential demand for such technology, currently paralleled by an increased willingness of practitioners to provide it. Finally, sex selection evidences the extreme polarization of public views developing in response to, rather than in anticipation of, the promise and threats such technology may offer and pose—creating an environment ripe for unwarranted, premature, and ultimately unconstitutional legislation.

Human history has long revealed a dramatic and undeniably prevalent human desire to control the future, development, and even traits of children. Children have occupied a common and central role in the lives of adults both through time and across races, and the longevity of parent-child relationships, in many cultures, is perhaps unique in the animal kingdom. Most adults feel the biological drive (and often religious obligation) to replicate, and carry a strong commitment to raise their children. Since children become so great a focus of parental intent, purpose, and even meaning, it is thus not surprising that parents seek to influence their development. It is equally unsurprising, given humankind's irrepressible desire to impose order in life, find meaning behind seeming chaos, and harness nature's forces, that men and women have continually sought keys to creation itself.

Sex selection is just one context in which this desire has frequently inspired direct action. Through the passing centuries, people have unrelentingly pursued and practiced techniques believed to influence the sex of children. Methods fanciful, cruel, and bizarre evidence the depth and breadth of the desire to do so. Infanticide was for millennia, and in some places remains, a successful (if inhumane) technique for eliminating a child to make room for another of the desired sex. From a coldly logical perspective, however, postconceptive techniques are strikingly inefficient since they typically eliminate the un-

> *"Studies have revealed an increasing willingness . . . to use sex selection procedures."*

wanted without actually providing the wanted. Consequently, the imaginative focused efforts primarily on preconceptive methods.

One might loosely term preconceptive methods of influencing the sex of a child as "biologic" or "symbolic." The biologic methods involve prescribed behavior during (or timing of) copulation or specific variations in the female diet. In contrast, symbolic methods are magical and mysterious.

Early biologic methods capitalized upon supposed correlations between offspring sex and the vigor of copulation, the side of the body providing the semen or egg, the method of breathing during orgasm, the timing of the female orgasm relative to that of the male, and even properly timed bites on a woman's ear. Some people even recommended raping one's wife to produce a male, on the theory that the more "male" a man acted, the greater the likelihood of fathering a boy. Dietetic theories also proliferated, culminating during the Middle Ages in more than a few women partaking in a ceremony involving the consumption of lion's blood, followed by copulation under a full moon while an abbot prayed for a child of the desired sex. Later dietetic theories extolled the role in sex selection of fish, seeds, sugars, peas, lettuce, cheese, salt, sweets, and even the testes of certain animals.

Early symbolic methods for preselecting sex correlated gender with the side of the bedpost on which one's trousers were hung, the maintenance of appropriate flowers in the windowsill, cross-dressing prior to intercourse, and prescribed songs sung (or objects taken) in bed.

> *"At least 70 clinics in the U.S. . . . offer sperm separation for the purposes of sex preselection."*

Because none of these methods proved particularly reliable, however, they stand more as a testament to frustrated and grasping demand than as an indication of a corresponding supply. That demand continues to this day. While it may not be as strong in the United States as it is in India or China, the demand is strong nonetheless. Studies of sex preferences in the United States, spanning over 50 years, reveal a continuing preference for a male child as the only child, or, alternatively, as the first child. A recent study of women alone, for example, indicated that they would prefer to birth 161 boys for every 100 girls in a one-child context. Similarly, their preferences would yield 171 to 100 first-born boys to girls in the multi-child context. Significantly, studies have revealed an increasing willingness to pursue and to use sex selection procedures.

The wide variety of reasons why people might prefer to have their next child be of one sex or another only contributes to the aggregation of demand. Individual parents may have "sequential" or "compositional" goals. Sequential goals concern preferences to have children of one sex *before* the other sex. Compositional goals concern the preferred ratio of sexes within the family. These latter goals may include the desire to have more, or to have exclusively, offspring of one sex, to complement a child of one sex with another of the other, or to have a child of a sex opposite to that shared by a string of children.

Parental preferences can span the spectrum of the fact-based, practical, stereotypical, and irrationally prejudiced. Parents' sequential or compositional goals may derive from associating with each sex different degrees of economic potential, status, or parentally desired personality and behavioral traits. Actual (or only subjectively perceived) superiority of boys, for example, in earning potential, or prevalence in girls, for example, of milder childhood demeanor, may affect the formulation of these goals. In other instances, parents may simply prefer the symmetry of having one child of each sex, or wish to diminish the chances of bearing a child with sex-linked diseases, such as Tay-Sachs disease, or more than 400 others.

Technology Makes Sex Preference Possible

As is now well-known, the egg, supplied by the female, always carries an X chromosome. A male's sperm carries either an X or Y chromosome. An egg fertilized by an X chromosome yields a girl; the Y chromosome leads to a boy. Since this was discovered in 1924, researchers have scrutinized human conditions and behavior for clues to controllable factors that might skew the sex ratio; sex selection research began in earnest.

Postconceptive techniques enable sex selection both *in vivo* (in the body) or *in vitro* (out of the body). Currently available *in vivo* techniques require discovery of the sex of a developing embryo or fetus (by ultrasound, chorionic villi sampling, or amniocentesis) and subsequent abortion if it is of the "wrong" (more accurately, "dispreferred") sex. Postconceptive *in vitro* techniques, in contrast, require the selection, and implantation in a woman, of one of several eggs fertilized in a laboratory.

Preconceptive techniques also may be *in vivo* or *in vitro*. Preconceptive *in vivo* theories prevalent today involve coital timing and manipulation of diet, hormones, and cervical mucus acidity. Preconceptive *in vitro* techniques require separation of X- from Y-bearing sperm, as much as possible, followed by artificial insemination of the woman using the "enriched" semen, in which the ratio of X- to Y-bearing sperm has been skewed in favor of the desired sex.

Methods for separating sperm, however, considerably antedated techniques for evaluating the success of those methods. Mass impregnation followed by observation of the sex ratio at birth, obviously, was and is rather impractical. But in 1964 a researcher developed a technique to stain Y-bearing sperm with a material that fluoresces under ultraviolet light, thereby enabling researchers to assess visually the success of various sperm-separation techniques. The promise offered by this evaluative technique spawned additional quests for sperm separation methods.

> *"Offspring trait selection . . . influences each individual human's reproductive success and inclusive fitness."*

With the 1971 discovery that the X-bearing sperm is 3% larger than the Y-bearing, and that the X-bearing swims more slowly (though further), researchers developed processes designed to separate sperm by size, weight, or motility. In the most successful technique, sperm is introduced to the top of a test tube containing three increasingly dense layers of the protein albumin. If a woman wants to conceive a boy (the method is rather less effective in selecting for girls) she is inseminated with the Y-enriched fluid from one end of the tube, to which the faster Y-bearing sperm have travelled.

While the method is not perfect, the most recent data indicate that the method can skew the probability of conceiving a boy from roughly 50% to approximately 72%. To put this in perspective, this would skew the sex ratio for selected offspring from roughly 1:1 to 3:1 if those employing the technique consistently selected for the same sex.

TST supply increases steadily. Studies now indicate that practitioners, many of whom were previously reticent to provide trait-selection services, are increasingly willing to supply sex selection procedures to those who request them. At least 70 clinics in the U.S., for example, already offer sperm separation for the purposes of sex preselection. Swiftly advancing TSTs afford increasing access to objects of longstanding desires. In addition to the sex selection methods described above, these technologies allow a woman, for example, to learn basic genetic information about the human embryo when it is only three days, that is *8 cells*, old. Such information may as easily reveal the sex as disclose the presence of genes coding for particular traits, deleterious or otherwise.

> *"Access to TST should be considered as protected a liberty as is access to*

Demand, supply, and a concomitant market are generally not problematic (at least in the short term) so long as private desires confront only public acquiescence. But in sex selection, as with trait-selection and technologically facilitated reproduction in general, beliefs frequently run strong—and at odds with each other. With increased public discourse in the social science and medical literature, positions have become increasingly polarized, with diminishing numbers of neutral observers. While some have argued eloquently for nearly blanket reproductive freedom, others have begun extensive calls for the outright prohibition of sex selection through criminal and civil penalties. Two such state prohibitions have already been passed. . . .

Reproductive Strategies

The pressures of natural selection ensure that some methods of reproduction, in average situations, will succeed better than others and that similar methods may require significantly varying reproductive strategies.

Some creatures, for example, lay eggs while others give birth to live young. Of those that lay eggs, some protect them (like most birds), and others do not (like most fish). Those species not laying eggs evidence a wide variety of characteristics in gestation period, number of offspring, developmental stage of offspring at birth, duration of adult care, and age of reproductive maturity. Thus creatures nearer the bottom of the food chain and more heavily subject to predation, like rabbits, tend to have greater numbers of offspring over their reproductive years while those at the higher end, like humans, tend to have fewer. In general, the less parental care there is, the more offspring are produced and the greater is the infant and juvenile mortality. In any event, natural selection is more "concerned" with how many survive to reproductive age than it is with how many are initially born.

Together, these principles make evident that natural selection operates inexorably, over passing millennia, upon variations of genetically passed traits, whether physical or behavioral. Natural selection thereby affects the reproductive strategies, and hence inclusive fitness, of each individual reproducing creature on the planet. Each of them, like it or not, has its gene lines subject to the patiently pruning test of reproductive success.

Consequently, offspring trait selection, by any means whatever, influences each individual human's reproductive success and inclusive fitness. Its direct and profound impact upon reproductive success suggests that if we in fact value reproductive autonomy in the ways the Supreme Court has articulated, then to be consistent access to TST should be considered as protected a liberty as is access to abortion procedures.

Sex Selection as Reproductive Strategy

To explore what this means in a concrete example, consider the evidence indicating that sex selection may be part of an adaptive reproductive strategy.

The Trivers-Willard Model: Sex Selection Can Be a Component of an Adaptive Reproductive Strategy Sex itself is merely one adaptive variation of reproductive traits; it is not necessary for reproduction. Not all species exhibit sexual dimorphism, like humans. Some species have no sex, some have thirteen, and individuals in other species are hermaphroditic, containing fully functional male *and* female organs. In fact a variety of creatures change from one sex to another depending on environmental conditions. The existence and role of different sexes in reproduction is, itself, a part of a reproductive strategy. So, too, is the method of sexual differentiation in offspring. For an assortment of fish, reptiles, worms, and plants, for example, the sex of embryonic young can be determined by temperature.

Since even minor differences between individuals may affect inclusive fitness, it follows that such major differences as the "whether" and "which" of sex may result in the divergence of reproductive strategies. The effect of sex on inclusive fitness obviously includes the effects of *offspring* sex. Consequently, one might predict that the ability to influence or skew the sex ratio of offspring would be, in certain circumstances, an evolutionarily adaptive trait. In 1973 two evolutionary biologists so predicted (in the later-termed "Trivers-Willard Model"), creating an uproar. There is now substantial evidence, however, (much of it compiled by former critics now converted), that the Model accurately fits observations, and has relevance to human reproduction.

The Trivers-Willard Model predicts that if the condition of mothers during the period of parental investment correlates with the probable reproductive success of their offspring, natural selection should favor the ability of parents to adjust their investment in the sexes to favor the sex with the best reproductive prospects.

> *"[Poor] women . . . are more likely to breast-feed their daughters than their sons."*

To see why this is so, imagine a population of caribou in which the physical condition of adult females varies from good to poor as indicated, for example, by weight. Assume that a female in good condition is better able to raise her calf than is a female in poor condition, so that at the end of the period of caregiving (or "parental investment"), the healthiest and strongest calves will tend to be the offspring of the adult females who were in the best condition during the caregiving period.

Assume further that some tendency exists for the differences in the condition of calves at the end of that period to be maintained into adulthood. Finally, assume that such adult differences in condition affect male reproductive success more strongly than they affect that of females. That is, assume that male caribou in good condition tend to exclude other males from breeding, thereby inseminating many more females themselves, while females in good condition, through their greater ability to invest in their young, show only a moderate increase in repro-

> *"Much human reproductive behavior reflects the attempt to vindicate biological, genetic self-interest."*

ductive success. Under these assumptions, an adult female in good condition who produces a son will leave more surviving "grandchildren" than a similar female who produces a female offspring—while an adult female in poor condition who produces a female offspring will leave more surviving "grandchildren" than a similar female who produces a male. Over time, then, the pressure of natural selection would favor a randomly generated but genetically inheritable trait enabling a female to produce more males when she is in good condition and females when she is in poor condition.

Sustained and wide-ranging sex ratio research over the last twenty years tends to confirm the Trivers-Willard Model. Animals as diverse as red deer, opossums, coypu, lemmings, jewel wasps, spider monkeys, and rhesus macaques all support the proposition that a female increases her inclusive fitness by skewing the sex ratio of offspring toward one sex or another, as her own condition deviates from the average adult physical and social condition. While it is sometimes unclear whether a given animal skews sex ratio by differential implantation or abortion in the womb, by sex-preferential care or infanticide, or by some combination of these, the evidence to date indicates that the ability and predisposition to do so is genetically inheritable and, in fact, often a superior reproductive strategy to one that is sex-neutral.

Evolutionary Biology in the Human Context: Sex Selection

One cannot determine with precision the extent to which a given behavior is genetically suggested, culturally learned, or the product of an identifiable combination of the two. But it is the net long-term effect of reproductive strategies, rather than the proximate cause, that is relevant for our purposes. These effects significantly affect an individual's reproductive success, and any governmental influence over them may thus implicate an individual's most basic decisions about parenting and reproduction. Consequently, governmental impediments will raise constitutional concerns.

Many adaptive strategies may have arisen either by biology or through learned behavior. In some cultures, for example, it is considered legitimate for a man to order the death of children a new wife has borne by union with a prior mate. In other cultures, as is widely known in anthropological circles, there is a strong association across human cultures between the incidence of extra-marital sex and the propensity of men to favor with resources their sister's sons, to whom they are likely to be more related genetically than they are to the sons of their wives. While one cannot prove that all reproductive strategies are evolutionarily adaptive, many do fit the natural selection model.

More relevant to this analysis is the evidence that the Trivers-Willard Model has probative significance in the context of human reproduction. Application of the model to humans is complicated by the tendency for males to invest parental effort in their young (rather than primarily spreading sperm as widely as possible), which diminishes the variance in male reproductive success. And, obviously, we would expect further deviation from the Model due to the increased cognitive and emotional capacities our species typically exhibits. Nevertheless, much evidence indicates that the contrasting reproductive potentials of the two sexes frequently results, even in humans, in the differential rearing of children in accordance with a mother's physical, economic, and social condition. At the moment, such differential rearing in the human context appears to be somewhat more the product of differential investment of parental resources, rather than of a skew in the sex ratio at birth. Nonetheless, a body of evidence exists to support even the latter conclusion, and the fact that humans already have some

"Trait selection . . . has already found expression in other creatures and, it appears, in humans."

capability (albeit an unconscious one) to skew the offspring sex ratio is obvious from the sex ratio at birth, which exhibits a steady skew toward 105:100 boys to girls.

But the differential rearing does fit the Trivers-Willard Model's prediction that when, for a given amount of parental investment, sons in good condition will out-reproduce their sisters, and daughters in poor condition will out-reproduce their brothers in poor condition, sons should be favored by parents with much to invest, and daughters by parents with little. The imbalanced childhood sex ratio of the Mukogodo of central Kenya, for example, fits the Model. Mukogodo men are poor and low status relative to men from neighboring groups, and have difficulty finding mates. They thus have significantly poorer reproductive prospects than Mukogodo women, who may marry either Mukogodo men, or those from wealthier neighbor groups. The Model predicts that Mukogodo couples should favor daughters since they have better reproductive prospects than sons. In fact, the childhood sex ratio (ages 0–4) is significantly female-biased. Girls outnumber boys 100 to 67. On the island of Ifaluk in the Western Pacific husbands of high traditional and salaried status and their wives do in fact spend much more time and energy on sons than do parents without such status, who tend to spend much more time and energy on daughters.

Women in the United States with annual household incomes of less than $10,000, or without an adult male present to share parental investment, are more likely to breast-feed their daughters than their sons. Moreover, women without an adult male present also tend to breast-feed their daughters more than five months longer than the sons they do breast-feed (consonant with the prevailing practice among Mukogodo women). And a recent study of modern testators in Vancouver revealed a pattern consistent with that which has emerged both across time and among various cultures: wealthy parents favored sons in their wills—whereas those with small estates discriminated against them.

TSTs Deserve Heightened Scrutiny

What should we do with all this information on biology, history, activity, and conflict? First, we can see sex selection as simply a paradigm of ways in which much human reproductive behavior reflects the attempt to vindicate biological, genetic self-interest. Human reproductive strategies include trait selection in offspring, which itself may involve, without being limited to, manipulation of offspring sex ratio. Sex selection also presents an example of trait selection that has already found expression in other creatures and, it appears, in humans; it has a pervasive history in cultures spanning the planet. . . .

Technologies that do and will facilitate the selection of certain traits in children are undeniably and powerfully disturbing. Initial indicators, such as legislation prohibiting sex selection in the abortion context, suggest that states may try to prohibit or regulate some or all TSTs. Evolutionary biology can prove useful when considering the legal and policy implications of such acts.

Evolutionary biology provides powerful new insights that more completely inform the contemporary concept of human reproduction. One can never logically conclude, of course, that such insights into the way something is, without more, speak meaningfully to the way something ought to be. Such a conclusion requires reference to existing or emerging value systems. However, the Supreme Court has already usefully articulated, in a line of cases currently culminating with *Planned Parenthood v. Casey*, important legal and social values that inform our laws and policies governing, and at times protecting, our reproductive behavior. The standard *Casey* articulates, namely that laws interfering with reproductive matters involving the most basic decisions that a person can make about parenting and family must be subjected to heightened and probing judicial scrutiny, applies squarely to TSTs.

> *"Attempting to select offspring traits will . . . represent one of the most basic decisions about parenting."*

While the boundaries of reproductive autonomy are not completely clear, evolutionary biology makes plain that offspring trait-selection has enormous genetic import and commensurate consequence to individual inclusive fitness. It has long been, and will continue to be, a fundamental influence on biological destiny. Because attempting to select offspring traits will therefore and necessarily represent one of the most basic decisions about parenting, family, and reproduction that an individual may make in her lifetime, consistency requires that these attempts should be subject to the same federal protection as that afforded abortion by *Casey*.

Chapter 5

What Would Be the Effect of Regulating Reproductive Technologies?

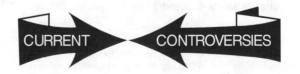

Regulation of Reproductive Technologies: An Overview

by Shannon Brownlee

About the author: *Shannon Brownlee is a senior editor for* U.S. News & World Report, *a weekly newsmagazine.*

A couple would have to want a baby very badly to go through what Irene and Peter R. did to have their son, Sam. Married at 33, Irene and Peter tried for two years to conceive before going to the first of a string of fertility specialists. That was in 1986, the beginning of a six-year, $100,000 medical odyssey that took them to fertility clinics in New York, London, Houston, Austin, Los Angeles and San Francisco and subjected Irene to five emotionally traumatic and sometimes physically painful attempts at in vitro fertilization (IVF). Sam was born after Irene's sixth IVF. His sister, Hannah, was born more than a year later after another $10,000 IVF procedure. Peter expresses no regrets as he strokes his son's head: "I'd rather have kids than the money."

The Fertility Business

So, apparently, would a lot of couples. While few are willing—or able—to go to the same extremes that Irene and Peter did, Americans spent $2 billion in 1994 in their quest for a child, and the baby-making business is booming. There were 30 fertility clinics in America in 1985; now there are more than 300, several of which are run by a publicly traded corporation. The potential market for their services is substantial. According to the National Center for Health Statistics, the overall rate of infertility has remained constant since 1965, but the aging of the massive baby boom generation has caused the sheer number of infertile couples to swell to 2.3 million. Infertility among couples between the ages of 35 and 44 is on the rise.

But unlike Irene and Peter, the vast majority of couples—about three quarters—walk out of fertility centers empty-handed. At best, high-tech baby making is an imperfect science. At worst, it is an unregulated industry that critics charge takes advantage of desperate couples. "The problem with this field is that patients don't realize it's a business," says Jonathan Van Blerkom, co-director of Reproductive Genetics In Vitro, a Denver clinic.

The fertility business has operated virtually without federal rules since 1979, when the government banned federally funded embryo research. Now, clinics have begun to respond to a law enacted in 1992 that required clinics to keep uniform success statistics, report them and submit to an accreditation process. But the minimal oversight will do little to improve the success rates at the worst clinics, leaving it to couples to separate the truth from the hype. In the worst cases, they run up huge bills in repeated and futile attempts to get pregnant. "I've seen people mortgage their homes and go into debt trying to have a baby," says Nancy DiVestea, co-president of the Washington, D.C., chapter of RESOLVE, an organization for helping infertile couples cope.

Even the most well-informed couples can find it difficult to imagine how emotionally and physically draining the high-tech baby chase can be. A woman begins a typical course of treatment with injections of powerful hormone-regulating drugs, which first depress her monthly cycle, sending her into instant, temporary menopause and sometimes plunging her into an emotional tailspin. Other drugs then stimulate her ovaries to ripen an average of a dozen eggs. If a woman's ovaries respond to this boost—and many do not—her doctor uses ultrasound and blood tests to judge the moment when the eggs are ripe and then extracts them with a long needle inserted through the vaginal wall. The eggs are mixed in a petri dish with the husband's sperm, and the resulting embryos are incubated for three days. Finally, the embryos, each consisting of only a few cells, are inserted into the woman's uterus.

The Percentages of Success

IVF offers an average take-home baby rate of 17 percent, with figures higher or lower depending on the age of the woman, the procedure and the clinic. A *U.S. News* analysis of most recent data from the American Society for Reproductive Medicine for 172 clinics shows that the chances of bringing home a baby for women under the age of 39 were 19 percent on average in 1992. Fertility dropped dramatically to an average of 6.6 percent for women 40 and older. By comparison, the odds that fertile couples will conceive in any month are only 20 percent. The clinics' track records vary widely. Some reported success rates as high as 50 percent while others did not produce a single child.

"The baby-making business is booming."

Even a slim chance seems better than none to couples who have tried everything to conceive. In 1988, 1.4 million women sought fertility services. In 1992, about 37,000 women went the high-tech route, but only 5,556 were rewarded with babies. In spite of the long odds, the hardest part for many couples is knowing when to stop. After three major pelvic surgeries, Linda DeBenedictis, a teacher in Boston, and her husband, John, began IVF in 1985. On their first two attempts, John's sperm failed to fertilize Linda's eggs. "We were devastated," Linda recalls. Her eggs were fertilized on the third and fourth tries, but Linda failed to get pregnant. They attempted GIFT (for gamete intrafallopian transfer), the latest trend in fertility treatments, and then another IVF. After six years and a total of 11 high-tech attempts, the couple had spent $40,000 of their own money along with thousands more paid for by insurance. "I've thought about adoption," says Linda, "but I can't imagine one more disappointment."

Persistence

Clinics do not make it easy for patients to step off the baby merry-go-round. Couples sit in waiting rooms decorated with pictures of babies conceived through the clinic; their doctors tell them that persistence pays off. Libby Carr, a Canton, Mass., schoolteacher, believed she would be among the lucky ones for six years, until she and her husband, Kevin, finally gave up on IVF and adopted a boy. "'It doesn't always work the first time. Don't give up.' Even the nurses tell you that," Carr recalls. "They tell you about someone who had gone through it 10 times and it finally worked. They give you the feeling that no matter what the percentage is, for you it will work out."

In fact, persistence pays off only rarely. Clinics typically tell patients their chances of conception are the same for each IVF attempt, up to about four tries, after which pregnancy rates drop. But a 1992 study

> *"The fertility business has operated virtually without federal rules since 1979."*

by Edward Kaplan, a professor of management sciences at Yale, showed that the chances of pregnancy fall after the first unsuccessful try. Of 571 women who started treatment at Yale's infertility center, 13 percent got pregnant on the first attempt, 10.7 percent on the second try, 6.9 percent by the third go-round, and only 4.3 percent by the fourth.

Kaplan suspects that the few women who are going to get pregnant do so within the first two or three tries; for most of the rest, continuing is almost futile, a fact that doctors and patients evade by focusing on new developments. "You try never to tell a patient that it's hopeless," says Barbara Weiss, of the Women's Medical Group in Santa Monica, Calif. "Every few years they come up with something new."

Critics charge that part of the reason it's hard to tell patients to stop is that clinics need the business. Fertility centers have proliferated because the profit potential is high and start-up costs are not. According to Richard Blackham, chief operating officer for Reproductive Genetics In Vitro, it costs about $500,000 to set up a free-standing fertility clinic. A staff of six runs another $500,000 a year, including a reproductive endocrinologist, whose income averages about $260,000, an embryologist, who makes about $100,000, and various technicians. A single IVF procedure, ordinarily the least expensive of the high-tech options, brings in between $5,000 and $15,000, with an additional $2,000 for fertility drugs. Other more expensive fertility procedures can command as much as $20,000, including drugs. "Whether you do 10 cycles a month or 1,000, the setup costs are the same and the break-even point is 10 women a month," says Barry Behr, an embryologist at Stanford Medical Center's infertility clinic who worked for eight years in private clinics. "After that, it's gravy."

> *"Even a slim chance seems better than none to couples who have tried everything to conceive."*

Yet only a fifth of the nation's clinics treat more than 10 patients a month because there simply aren't enough paying customers to go around, despite the large potential market. To stay profitable, clinics must recruit patients. Geoffrey Sher, who has one of the highest success rates in the business, says two-thirds of the 1,000 procedures a year performed by the four California Pacific Fertility Center clinics, of which he is executive medical director, are part of "discount packages"—such as a one-time $13,000 fee covering up to three IVF cycles. His staff includes a full-time marketing professional, and the four clinics sponsor seminars, a newsletter and radio ads. Sher is unapologetic about his tactics. "We're not saying to people, 'Have IVF when you don't need it,'" he says. "We're saying, 'If you need IVF, look at us.'"

Pushing Expensive Treatments

Fertility centers affiliated with hospitals have also become aggressive advertisers. "The patient has to come back to deliver the baby," says Gil Mileikowsky, a Los Angeles fertility specialist. "So the hospital carries a very positive aura, with a large referral potential." The pressure to recruit patients can be particularly keen for big clinics. Carl Herbert, a doctor who once worked at a large fertility clinic, says that "big clinics have leveraged themselves like a big business to make a big profit. When you're so leveraged, it puts pressure on you to treat your patients as potential income rather than individualizing their care."

Such pressures can also lead clinics to push patients into more expensive, high-tech procedures before trying less expensive methods first. During their initial visit to a Virginia clinic, one Washington, D.C., couple was urged to try GIFT, at a cost of $12,000. After a second opinion, the wife is now undergoing intrauterine insemination, or IUI, for $280. Other doctors continue performing useless procedures because insurance will pay. Behr recalls treating a woman who had undergone 17 IUIs, although the chances of pregnancy fall to zero after the fourth attempt with this procedure. The woman got pregnant with her first IVF.

Some clinics are quick to trumpet their successes with cutting-edge tech-

153

niques, and the media often willingly oblige with uncritical stories. In January 1994, for example, the *Rocky Mountain News* reported that two women had delivered babies thanks to "assisted hatching," an experimental technique using acid to dissolve a tiny hole in the embryo's outer coat. At the time, William B. Schoolcraft, medical director of the Center for Reproductive Medicine in Denver, where the procedure was performed, claimed an "unofficial" success rate of 62 percent, a number many fertility specialists find astonishing. Schoolcraft was quoted as saying that hatching is "the biggest fertility development in five years." Schoolcraft now says the clinic has a 55 percent rate over two years. Yet at least one case of hatching has resulted in conjoined—or Siamese—twins, an exceedingly rare defect, and there are rumors of other cases.

The result of the media's focus on gee-whiz technology is customers who demand the very latest breakthrough and clinic directors who feel compelled to offer it—whether or not the technique has been proven safe or effective. A new method for treating male infertility called ICSI (for intracytoplasmic sperm injection) provides a case in point. ICSI shot to prominence shortly after its introduction to the United States from Belgium in 1993, when it was touted on the television newsmagazine and talk-show circuit. NBC's Maria Shriver dubbed it "a bold new advance [that] is giving babies to couples who tried everything but failed."

Now, some fertility specialists are speculating that ICSI will one day replace conventional IVF, even though most women's eggs fertilize without it and little is known about the technique's long-term consequences. A surprising 40 percent of infertility is the man's problem, and men are partially to blame for another 20 percent of cases. One study in Belgium showed that 28 percent of women have "ongoing pregnancies" or have delivered babies through ICSI. Thus far, most ICSI babies have been born healthy. But with few animal studies to draw from, scientists must simply wait to see what the future holds for the children they help produce.

> *"Clinics do not make it easy for patients to step off the baby merry-go-round."*

That's not stopping couples from clamoring for the procedure. "Patients call up asking if you offer ICSI. If you don't, they go elsewhere," says Behr. Mastering ICSI takes a steady hand and practice. An embryologist uses a hand-crafted glass or stainless-steel needle to capture a single sperm, tail first. The needle then pierces the zona pellucida, the egg's protective coating, to deposit the captive sperm in the egg's core—all done through a microscope. In Behr's view, such high-tech procedures should be performed only by a few fertility centers that specialize in them. "If you needed brain surgery, your general practitioner wouldn't offer to do it," he says.

There is little agreement in the field about how to end abuses—or even that abuses still exist. One solution in the eyes of some fertility specialists, as well as many patients, is insurance coverage. Insurance would almost certainly bring costs down. Seven states now mandate coverage, while most insurers in the rest of the country refuse to pay for fertility treatments, lumping them in the same class of nonvital procedures as tummy tucks and hair transplants. Without in-surers to haggle over prices, both pharmaceutical manufacturers and fertility clinics have been free to raise their rates. For example, in 1984 the price of Pergonal, a common fertility drug, was $12 an am-

"Fertility centers affiliated with hospitals have also become aggressive advertisers."

pul; now it's as much as $65 in the United States—and $17 just across the bor-der in Mexico. In 1989, the cost of IVF was $3,000 less than it is now. But in Massachusetts, where insurers have been required by law to pay for fertility treatments since 1990, the average cost of IVF is $5,500, well below the price in most major metropolises.

But if Massachusetts's experience is any indication, insurance coverage would do little to improve success rates. Massachusetts clinics are no better at getting women pregnant than those in the rest of the country. Three quarters of the patients at Boston IVF, at Beth Israel Hospital, are covered by insurance, and in 1992, the clinic performed a whopping 1,288 egg retrievals, 320 more than the next-busiest clinic in the country. Yet the clinic's success rate for women under 40 was only 10.5 percent, 6.5 percentage points lower than the average for all clinics. Selwyn Oskowitz, a director at Boston IVF, says one reason for its low rate is that the clinic does not turn away women who are "low responders," those who produce only an egg or two in response to hormonal stimulation. Although such women have only a 5 percent chance of success, says Oskowitz, "that's a tangible figure. Those are still beautiful babies."

Big Ticket

More than anything, mandated insurance coverage would provide the fertility industry with many more paying customers. Harley Earl, president and CEO of National Reproductive Medical Centers, which runs four California clinics, notes: "We're barely tapping the market." Insurance would change that. Blue Cross Blue Shield, which carries a third of the patients in Massachusetts, re-ports that payments for high-tech fertility treatments rose from $2 million in 1990 to $10 million in 1993.

Federal law now requires [as of 1995] the industry to keep standardized records of all procedures, which many already report to the American Society for Reproductive Medicine voluntarily. The law also requires clinics to be ac-credited and their lab procedures monitored by the Centers for Disease Control and Prevention, in Atlanta. But it's unclear how the CDC will carry out Congress's wishes because it got "zero money" from Congress for the new task, says James Marks, director of the CDC's division of reproductive health.

Even more than federal oversight, what the fertility industry needs is some good science. "This field hasn't attracted many high-caliber people," says Van Blerkom, who consulted for the National Institutes of Health panel that set guidelines for future human embryo research. In its rush to embrace the newest technology, the industry has failed to determine whether each new advance was actually an improvement. For example, GIFT and ZIFT (for zygote intrafallopian transfer) are performed widely, though they require surgery and cost nearly twice as much as IVF. Now that clinical trials have finally been conducted, it turns out that ZIFT and possibly GIFT are no better than IVF. Even IVF itself may not be necessary in many cases: One Canadian study found that 8 percent of IVF candidates who simply waited six months got pregnant on their own.

Van Blerkom would like to see an impartial panel set up to assess both the safety and efficacy of the fertility industry. One vital task, for example, is to run studies to test suspicions that there might be a link between prolonged use of fertility drugs and ovarian cancer, a rare but mostly fatal malignancy.

Multiple Births

Another problem in the fertility industry that needs attention is the frequency of multiple births. *U.S. News*'s analysis of the 1992 clinic data reveals that more than half the 5,400 IVF babies came as part of a multiple birth. Such births are common because fertility doctors transfer numerous embryos to a woman's womb to boost her chances of pregnancy. (Only 2 percent of babies born to the general population are multiples.) Having multiple births is risky to both mother and offspring—and it is expensive. The average child born in a set of twins runs up $39,000 in hospital costs alone—10 times the average for a singleton. Multiples are 10 times more likely than singletons to be born prematurely and at low birth weight, and they appear to be at a higher risk for birth defects. A study in the *British Medical Journal* found that cerebral palsy occurred 47 times more often in triplets and 8 times more in twins than singletons. Most clinics now restrict the number of embryos they transfer, but the high incidence of multiples can be avoided if the industry is willing to move more slowly and test each new procedure before putting it into practice.

Still, even the industry's sharpest critics do not want to see it shut down. "There is a wonderful side to all of this," says Van Blerkom. "Women are having babies. But you want to make sure you do no harm." As the fertility business gallops along, it is leaving society to face a host of medical and ethical dilemmas. In 1993, researchers created multiple copies of a single embryo, evoking the specter of a woman giving birth to identical children many years apart. Almost every month, yet another menopausal woman gives birth to a child, thanks to the technology that allows a younger woman's eggs to be inserted into the womb of

"There is little agreement in the field about how to end abuses."

156

another. One day it may be technically feasible to extract the immature eggs from a female fetus, grow them in the lab and then implant them into an infertile woman. The medical miracle of helping a couple conceive has been irreversibly transformed into a business. Until it begins policing itself, says California fertility doctor Arthur Wisot, "this is a situation where the consumer has to kick the tires."

Reproductive Technologies Must Be Regulated to Protect Society

by Marvin F. Milich

About the author: *Marvin F. Milich is an assistant professor of business law at Queens College of the City University of New York.*

The arrival of the first human conceived *in vitro*, Louise Brown, on July 25, 1978, made the public acutely aware that new reproductive technologies would change social and legal familial relationships. The emergence of these new technologies will have a profound effect on the male-female association so dominant in Western culture. The question, however, remains: to what extent will technological developments change the face of social and legal relationships among all interested parties?

With the prospect for the development of *in vitro* fertilization (IVF) technology, Aldous Huxley's vision in *Brave New World* could now conceivably become a reality—a world in which family relationships are replaced by "hatcheries," where embryos are produced and monitored in an artificial environment, where abolition of the family is followed by complete sexual freedom, and where reproduction is handled by the state. [As stated in the *St. Louis University Law Journal*,] "In Huxley's society, this life creating method was the major instrument of social stability because it enabled society to create standardized machine-minders for standardized machines. . . . Yesterday's science fiction, however, [has become] today's reality.". . .

The Interplay of Reproductive Technology and Legislative Solutions

Reproductive policy is inextricably linked to social values. As a result, as help for infertility is increasingly sought and reproductive technology makes further advances, greater problems will arise if they are not addressed as soon

Excerpted from "In-Vitro Fertilization and Embryo Transfer: Medical Technology + Social Values = Legislative Solutions" by Marvin F. Milich, *University of Louisville Journal of Family Law*, vol. 30, no. 4, 1991–92. Reprinted with permission.

as possible. While reproductive issues are politically taboo, the mere "[a]wareness of the existence of the problem in and of itself is not an assurance that the problem [will] be put on the 'public agenda,'" as R. Blank states. However, it is also clear that

> [b]ecause of the delicate moral and ethical issues raised, the temptation to refrain from any legislation . . . is strong. . . . [T]he absence of any consensus as to the propriety of the procedure indicates the need for some general guidelines. Otherwise, the procedures will be controlled only by the individual consciences of participants with no guaranteed protection for the resulting child and for society.

In the face of the foregoing dilemma, Blank notes that "[t]he heightened sensitivity to the social implications of genetic and reproductive technological development . . . and the heightened fear by some that societal decisions are being made without adequate public input have produced a growing concern over the question of who should control the critical policy decisions which face us." It is also clear in our society that public opinion carries considerable political weight on issues of concern to a large sector of the population. The unique problem with reproductive issues is that they directly affect a large part of society, generating a united public opinion about technology that affects the religious and ethical values we hold. In any case, the public alone cannot create reproductive policy.

> *"These new technologies will have a profound effect on the male-female association."*

Medical Information

Part of the equation also includes making the medical community more responsible for the advancement of reproductive technology within our society. A doctor can do a number of things to inform the prospective IVF patient. IVF practitioners should be required to do the following: (1) inform the individual patient as to statistical information about his or her center and other centers throughout the community and country regarding success rates and other medically pertinent information; (2) use the practical experience of treating patients as a mechanism to improve the quality and efficiency of his or her own center and other centers with the goal of making IVF treatment as pleasant and safe as possible to the oft times desperate patient; and (3) create a network among IVF practitioners that provides for a better flow of information and a way for doctors to communicate and shape the future of IVF and other reproductive technologies. . . .

Knowledgeable Patients

Another part of the solution to the sparsity of action on IVF is increased responsibility on behalf of the IVF patient. In a society that considers technology its greatest asset, we often develop a complacence toward technological advances because we rely so frequently on their use. In the area of reproductive technology, that sense of confidence is acutely necessary, yet a serious danger. Patients should look at IVF as a cure for infertility and not as an everyday convenience. In effect, [as an Illinois statute states], we must resist "the urge to deify IVF."

> *"Aldous Huxley's vision in* **Brave New World** *could now conceivably become a reality."*

In addition, prospective patients ought to be concerned with collecting and evaluating the information distributed by the physician. Part of resisting the deification of IVF should be to break down the "paternalistic model of interaction with physicians" [Illinois statute]. This can be best achieved through the implementation of the suggestions above regarding the publication of medical information and physician-patient interaction. If we promote these ideas, perhaps the public will become more aware of the objective—recognizing the seriousness of the need for regulation of IVF and prompting legislative action.

Finally, patients should know that there are recommended qualifications in place that serve as a bellwether for prospective IVF patients. Andrea Bonnicksen suggests that a woman with a good chance of success possess the following traits:

(1) between 25 and 34 years old;

(2) at an established center with multiple births;

(3) only one or two unsuccessful IVF attempts;

(4) husband with high sperm count; and

(5) tubal infertility with no other problems.

Blank would add the following to the list:

(1) couples must be legally married and in excellent health; and

(2) the menstrual cycle must be regular, the uterus and the ovaries normal and accessible to laparoscopy.

In sum, the patient should treat the IVF procedure with profound respect, being careful not to deify it. The operation should not be used as a novelty and should be understood to be the final effort for an infertile couple to give birth to their own child.

Responsible Government

Before suggesting some proposals for regulating IVF, some general comments are in order. First, much of the IVF debate seems to be caught up in the fiery political discourse now raging over abortion. The suggestion, then, that IVF policy should be set in the interest of clinical practice and in the interest of patients and away from embryo issues is a positive step toward a solution. Bonnicksen suggests that the most practical and effective way of achieving this goal is to encourage privatization of IVF with an eye toward self-monitoring.

This will aid in the policy objectives stated with regard to patients, physicians and the public.

This privatization will provide larger advantages. It will allow state legislatures to develop their own monitoring procedures, presumably based on a greater demand from the public for information due to a wider awareness of solutions for infertility. If this does not provide adequate monitoring, the state could respond with legislation covering every aspect of IVF, being careful, however, to meet constitutional guidelines. Further, the privatization will provide stability to the system. The state could provide regulations to govern centers and license the physicians that would streamline both the use and advance of IVF technology. In addition, government regulation has its own intrinsic value because it confers legitimacy on the direction of IVF. With no further ado, the following are my proposals for IVF regulation.

First, there is a need for a clearinghouse for information regarding IVF. The clearinghouse could gather information now required by federal regulation and publish regular reports with an eye toward encouraging private organizations to engage in IVF practice. Second, insurance companies should provide coverage for those who choose to engage in IVF activities. A number of states have already passed legislation to make insurance cover such practices. This type of legislation encourages the privatization movement.

On another level, there are a number of proposals that can be made to help IVF practice become safer, more efficient and more accessible. A primary suggestion would be to ensure that: (1) the gametes would be those of husband and wife only; (2) embryo wastage is not significantly higher in IVF than in *in vivo* fertilization; (3) the likelihood of fetal abnormality is no greater than it is in normal procreation; and (4) there is no intention to abort if abnormality does occur.

These suggestions are those of Robert McCormick and would solve several different problem areas. Suggestion (1) would prohibit the use of IVF for unmarried couples. The Supreme Court is unlikely to use *Eisenstadt*, *Roe*, and *Carey* to extend fundamental right protection to unmarried couples, thereby allowing the states to regulate in this manner under the "rational relation" test. Suggestions (2) and (3) are presumably taken care of in the process itself, while (4) prevents the possibility of abuses by affluent couples.

> *"Reproductive policy is inextricably linked to social values."*

Since *Roe* protects the right of a woman to abort her fetus regardless of the health of the prospective child, suggestion (4) could also be modified to provide no "extraordinary" intention to abort based on abnormality.

Additional suggestions would address the various social concerns presented throughout this article. Since a constitutional right attaches only if a couple cannot conceive naturally, one suggestion includes the requirement that the couple be infertile. Another suggestion includes having the parents sign a form that declares them the legal parents upon birth (thus, preventing the breakdown of the family) and includes provisions for disposal of "discards" (presumably under *Roe*, solving the moral dilemma of challenges of infanticide from conservative groups). This could be done through the withholding of federal funds for noncompliance. A further suggestion includes establishing a minimum standard of care for physicians. This will facilitate proper medical procedure and provide for a sense of security and safety in the public about IVF.

> *"The public alone cannot create reproductive policy."*

As for the liability of practitioners, there should be a limit on the availability of legal redress. Such a proposal should include a cause of action against a practitioner upon a showing of lack of due care by the practitioner in the exercise of the process. The parents should be entitled to costs for treatment of the defective child and general damages for the child's pain and suffering.

Finally, it should be noted here that any proposal for legislation should consider three concerns: (1) will the law be obeyed; (2) is it enforceable against the disobedient; and (3) is it prudent to undertake enforcement in view of the possibility of harmful effects in other areas of social life?

The proposals set forth previously can assure affirmative answers to (1) and (2). As to question (3), perhaps George Orwell has the best answer:

> *Brave New World* presents a fanciful and somewhat ribald picture of a society, in which the attempt to recreate human beings in the likeness of termites has been pushed almost to the limits of the possible. That we are being propelled in the direction of *Brave New World* is obvious. But no less obvious is the fact that we can, if we so desire, refuse to cooperate with the blind forces that are propelling us.

Sound IVF policy will allow us to propel ourselves in the direction of our choice. We must work with those blind forces and incorporate them into an IVF policy framework for future generations.

Surrogacy Should
Be Regulated

by Keith J. Hey

About the author: *Keith J. Hey is a professor at Thomas M. Cooley Law School in Lansing, Michigan.*

Medical technology continues to amaze and intrigue society with seemingly unending advancements in the enhancement and extension of human life. Rarely, however, does medicine make substantial advances in the promotion of human life, or, for that matter in any other aspect of the field, without creating corresponding legal problems. Rather, almost any new medical development introduces additional complex legal and moral entanglements.

Perhaps no area of medical technology has raised, or continued to foster, more interest than those advances made in assisted conception and its legal progeny, surrogacy arrangements. The desire to propagate, to produce and raise genetically related human beings, is one of the most fundamental instincts of men and women. But, increasingly, this goal is frustrated as the number of individuals suffering from infertility continues to increase. It is estimated that over two and a half million couples in the United States are unable to conceive a child by natural intercourse due to a defect or deficiency in one or both of the partners. The defect may be genetic, caused by an accident, or otherwise stem from a myriad of causes in either the male or female partner.

Historically, adoption was the alternative for those couples unable to have children, but the length of time required for the regulatory process to function and the limited number of adoptable children, particularly newborn babies, has left a trail of disappointed couples. Moreover, the process of adoption generally involved a child bearing no genetic relationship to either of the adopting parents. Thus, the basic urge for a genetic connection within the parent-child relationship was still missing.

During the last quarter of the twentieth century medical technology has made a number of techniques available to individuals incapable of natural reproduc-

Excerpted from "Assisted Conception and Surrogacy—Unfinished Business" by Keith J. Hey, *John Marshall Law Review*, vol. 26, no. 4, 1993. Reprinted courtesy of The John Marshall Law School.

tion. The process of *in vitro* fertilization, perfected in the late 1970s, has been rapidly followed by developments allowing the cryopreservation of human reproductive elements and, later, the transfer of human embryos through uterine lavage and implantation. Other procedures such as gamete interfallopian transfer, zygote interfallopian transfer, and micromanipulation of sperm into ova also made genetic reproduction possible in previously difficult or seemingly impossible situations.

The increased use of assisted conception processes such as *in vitro* fertilization and its medical progeny also greatly increased the number of those resorting to surrogacy arrangements, those nonmedical agreements whereby a woman would agree to conceive and give birth to a child for another person. In a typical situation the surrogate would consent, generally in exchange for a substantial fee, to undergo artificial insemination, *in vitro* fertilization, or embryo transplantation, in order to carry the resulting fetus to term and surrender the child immediately following birth. The more widely used form of surrogacy, sometimes referred to as "partial surrogacy," would have the sperm provided by the rearing father and the child would be given up to the father and his wife. However, the sperm could also be provided by an anonymous donor. The egg as well could be provided by either the rearing mother or by the surrogate or by a third party donor. An arrangement under which neither of the intended parents is genetically related to the child may be referred to as a "full surrogacy." The ability of medical science to retrieve, store, and implant the life-initiating cells, coupled with the contractual surrogacy arrangement, has created a variety of combinations for gestational and genetic parents of children born as a result of the combination of such medical technology and legal procedures.

Does a "Right" Answer Exist?

Although medical science was developing the procedures enabling many individuals to consider assisted reproduction techniques and arrangements, the idea of producing a child through one of the assisted conception procedures was often challenged as being contrary to the ethical or religious beliefs of many individuals and couples. Beyond that issue, the idea of a woman agreeing in advance of her child's birth to go through the childbearing process and then surrender her child to another person or couple runs contrary to concepts of the family as perceived by many in today's society. The ever-expanding combination of assisted

"Almost any new medical development introduces additional complex legal and moral entanglements."

conception techniques and contractual surrogacy arrangements has created a raft of legal problems for the courts and legislatures, not merely in the United States but throughout the world. How should a society deal with these latest chapters in the continuing saga of assisted conception? Should *in vitro* fertilization, embryo transplantation, and other fertility techniques be regulated by society? Should surrogacy arrangements be condemned, condoned, or controlled? A study of legislation and court decisions in the United States, Great Britain, and Australia reflects a broad range of positions on assisted conception and surrogacy, sometimes presented in simplistic fashion and other times stated in varying degrees of sophistication. Which approach is the more appropriate? Is there a "right" answer?

It is the position of this author that the piecemeal attempts to resolve issues on assisted conception and surrogacy arrangements have merely touched the tip of the extremely sensitive and multifaceted problems created by these new reproductive technologies. A careful analysis of court decisions and enacted legislation in the United States, while inconsistent in results, reflects substantial consistency in the lack of understanding or mere avoidance of the interrelated problems inherent in assisted conception and its legal stepchild, the surrogacy arrangement. In many jurisdictions the paucity of laws to regulate assisted reproduction or surrogacy has the effect of merely moving the problem through the legal process one small piece at a time, much like a youth kicking a tin can down a country road. Reaction is highly selective, more often than not because the issue is being chosen by the confines of litigation or by public outcry. One or more elements within this complex problem initiated by new medical advances is supposedly resolved without addressing the entire problem. What is needed is a comprehensive analysis and statutory enactment

> *"Reproductive technology desperately needs a truly uniform code."*

covering all of the various medical and legal aspects of assisted conception and surrogacy arrangements. Similar to the need in the commercial law field almost a half century ago for enactment of a Uniform Commercial Code to consolidate and coordinate the various phases of commercial law, reproductive technology desperately needs a truly uniform code to provide guidance for individuals and institutions involved in the process, and, more particularly, to protect those voiceless infants who will be born by virtue of such technology and/or contractual arrangements. . . .

Analysis of Surrogacy Decisions and Legislation

An analysis of the limited number of decisions on surrogacy combined with the enacted and proposed legislation in the United States, England, and Australia produces a number of similar characteristics. First, although several legislative enactments declare all surrogacy arrangements to be void, the theme of the *Baby M* decision and most legislation in the United States strikes at the commercial and financial aspects of the arrangement. This same concern is found in Australia and Great Britain statutes. Accepting the premise for the moment that only commercial arrangements are to be voided or made criminal, then altruistic surrogacy arrangements are not to be condemned, but are they to be ignored? Any surrogacy arrangement has as its basic purpose the bringing of human life into existence, a life which otherwise would not be created. The impact upon all consenting parties is obviously critical and, if the arrangement falls apart for one or more of a variety of reasons, the state may be forced to become a reluctant participant in the aftermath. Guidelines must be enacted to provide basic areas of needed protection for all of the individuals involved in the non-commercial surrogacy. Parties to

> *"Provision must be made to clearly identify issues of paternity and support for any child born as a result of a surrogacy arrangement."*

such an altruistic arrangement do not lose the need for counseling and medical testing merely because the surrogate is not being compensated for her role.

The second and perhaps even more critical similarity in surrogacy legislation is found in the lack of any reference to issues concerning the child born in a surrogacy arrangement. Legislation or judicial decisions declaring the surrogacy contract to be void or criminalizing the transaction will no doubt deter most potential surrogacy participants, but others may still pursue such activities, whether for compensation or not. Provision must be made to clearly identify issues of paternity and support for any child born as a result of a surrogacy arrangement. The Uniform Status Act does deal with issues affecting the child but does so without connecting into the other aspects of assisted conception.

The third similarity, and unfortunately so, is that the majority of recent legislation refers only to surrogate mother contracts and does not speak to the many facets of artificial insemination, *in vitro* fertilization, or embryo transfer. Admittedly, procedures for assisting reproduction deal with medical technology rather than the more legalistic issues in surrogacy. This differentiation is sufficiently important so that issues relating to assisted conception could be handled in other legislative coverage. Support for this argument might be more forthcoming if legislation on the medical advancements involved in assisting conception was being promoted at the same time as the legislation on surrogacy contracts. Even so, the more logical approach would have legislation on the medical aspects of assisted conception include the continuum of surrogacy arrangements.

A Thorough Statutory Scheme

Statutory enactments on surrogacy arrangements should not be adopted in a vacuum; such legislation needs to be part of a thorough statutory scheme regulating both the medical technologies and the contractual aftermaths. The shortcoming of most surrogacy legislation has resulted from a myopic understanding and/or treatment of the medical procedures involved in enabling surrogacy arrangements to become available to the public. Medical technology provided the impetus; it was only through the success of artificial insemination, *in vitro* fertilization, and embryo transfer procedures that surrogacy arrangements became a viable alternative for couples or individuals otherwise not capable of genetic parenthood. . . .

A Lack of Legislation

The current legislative attempts to regulate surrogacy arrangements are inherently flawed. A raft of problems remain to be solved. Are all surrogacy arrangements to be condemned or only those in which a fee is paid? Is money the issue or is it society's concept of how a family should be formed? Should *in vitro* fertilization, for either single or married women, be allowed without genetic testing of the gametes and psychological evaluation of the surrogate? Should not all parties to the arrangement receive appropriate counseling and legal advice? These are just a few of the issues currently unanswered by the paucity of legislative and judicial pronouncements on assisted reproduction and surrogacy arrangements.

The medical procedures to aid human conception continue to become more and more sophisticated. States failing to respond to the medical advancements or which pass laws dealing with only one or more segments of the issue can expect the dike to leak elsewhere and in a more rapid fashion. The need is for comprehensive legislation to deal with the total spectrum of medical and legal aspects of assisted conception and surrogacy, including paternity and support issues. The child born in a surrogacy arrangement must be protected without regard to the validity of the contract; the adults in a disputed surrogacy arrangement may well be able to fend for themselves but not so the child. The emotional reaction to such arrangements, coupled with the sensationalism attached to several gone-wrong surrogacy contracts, cannot be completely ignored when these issues are considered but any statutory enactment must provide the breadth of coverage to protect all innocent parties to any assisted conception or surrogacy arrangement. . . .

The focal point for resolving assisted conception and surrogacy disputes at a policy level lies in the state capitols and not in the courts. An appropriate balance of legal authority would have the courts placing a judicial stamp of approval on arrangements made by consenting parties under provisions first articulated by the state legislatures. The judicial process is poorly equipped to deal with the comprehensiveness of conception and surrogacy problems. Thus, the courts often resort to questionable analogies in resolving the conflict. As Judge Radigan stated in the *Baby Girl L.J.* decision, matters of public policy should be resolved by the legislature and not by the courts.

> *"Current legislative attempts to regulate surrogacy arrangements are inherently flawed."*

We are now in a new generation of family development and identification.

Although adoption procedures will continue to provide one path for childless individuals and couples, a new and sometimes more promising path has been opened by medical technology. It remains for the law, more particularly the legislative process, to provide the appropriate legal guidance for that technology. Until comprehensive legislation deals with all of the intricate issues in facilitating reproduction and surrogacy, the courts will proceed to slowly and painfully resolve those issues in an ad hoc and unsystematic process. Without extensive uniform legislation, the conflicting views found in the limited number of state statutes and judicial decisions will continue to spawn new doubts and tribulations for individuals seriously interested in pursuing a surrogacy arrangement.

Slow Motion Feet

In the Australian case of *Mount Isa Mines, Ltd. v. Pusey*, Justice Windeyer referred to "[l]aw, marching with medicine but in the rear and limping a little." This comment appropriately identifies the approach now being used by the courts in resolving reproduction and surrogacy issues. The law is developing blisters on its slow motion feet in an attempt to keep pace with medical technology. It need not be so. Resolution of the matter calls for a clear understanding of the medical aspects of assisted reproduction, combined with the necessary regulations covering all of the technological facets and legal arrangements following the scientific advancements. The opportunity now exists to bring the law alongside assisted reproduction technology. Some jurisdictions have already begun to reduce the distance between the two. The next several years should resolve whether the lessons of the *Baby M* decision . . . have been taken to heart or whether the law on assisted reproduction and surrogacy will continue to "limp along in the rear" for another generation while medicine continues its dramatic surge into the twenty-first century.

Sperm Banks
Should Be Regulated

by Mary E. Guinan

About the author: *Mary E. Guinan is a physician and researcher with the Office of HIV/AIDS of the U.S. Centers for Disease Control and Prevention in Atlanta, Georgia.*

The report of seven cases of human immunodeficiency virus (HIV) infection in women who were artificially inseminated by donor is another landmark in the history of the HIV epidemic in North America. Details of the investigation reveal that the women had received semen from one of five donors subsequently found to be HIV infected. The women were inseminated at fertility centers between 1981 and 1985, before the first laboratory test for HIV was licensed and available in the United States. The tragedy of these cases is compounded by the fear that more have gone unrecognized. Not all recipients of the semen of the infected donors could be found and 30 recipients refused to be tested. These cases bring the total to 12 known cases of HIV infection in women from artificially inseminated donor semen, four in Australia, two in Canada, and six in the United States. Might there be others that are unrecognized, given that as many as a million donor inseminations may have occurred since the covert HIV epidemic began in the 1970s?

This case series represents the experience of fertility clinics in the early 1980s with high operating safety standards. These clinics had in place requirements to screen semen donors for sexually transmitted diseases, which were neither mandatory nor standard practice at the time. In 1983 L. Mascola et al raised the issue of screening semen donors for sexually transmitted diseases because it was not being done routinely. These clinics also kept good records and were able to track retrospectively which of their clients received potentially infected semen and which of their donors might have been the source of infection. Otherwise these cases may never have been linked definitively to the insemination procedure. Evidence shows that many independent practitioners neither

Excerpted from "Artificial Insemination by Donor: Safety and Secrecy" by Mary E. Guinan, *JAMA*, vol. 273 (March 15, 1995):890–91.

screened donors nor kept linkage records. In 1982 a physician used semen from an unscreened donor (later found to carry hepatitis B antigen) to inseminate several women, one of whom developed life-threatening hepatitis B. Physicians who obtained semen from sperm banks were not required to keep records of which semen was used for a specific patient. Therefore, if semen bank specimens were identified as possibly contaminated, as in this series, many recipients could not be warned of the risk.

> *"Is artificial insemination any safer? . . . The answer is definitely yes."*

Now, 10 to 14 years after these seven women were infected with a lethal virus, is artificial insemination any safer? From an infection point of view, the answer is definitely yes. The risk of transmitting HIV or any infection during artificial insemination by donor is very low. In 1988 the Centers for Disease Control with the endorsement of the American Fertility Society, the American Academy of Obstetricians and Gynecologists, and the American Association of Tissue Banks issued the following recommendations for screening semen donors to prevent HIV infection. Donors should be screened for HIV antibody on the day of semen donation. The semen should be frozen and not used until the donor is tested again 6 months later and found to be HIV antibody-negative. This practice will prevent the use of semen from men who at the time of donation have early HIV infection but are HIV antibody-negative. The 6-month waiting period is a net that maximizes the safety.

Identities of Recipients, Donors Unknown

Safety loopholes still exist, which are complicated by the desire for secrecy, especially by the recipients and donors. Practitioners of artificial insemination are not required to register, and special training or licensing is not required. Therefore, it is difficult to monitor adherence to standard safety practices. With the exception of fertility clinics that offer the service, it is largely unknown who is practicing insemination. Despite the requirement by many states that artificial insemination be performed by a physician, a movement for "demedicalization" of insemination has become evident. Self-insemination by women who obtain sperm from various sources is not uncommon. In fact, a popular book on parenting for lesbians assumes that pregnancy will occur through self-insemination. It is argued that the success of these efforts testifies to the fact that no medical experience is necessary. What is of great concern is the infection risk of self-insemination if semen donors are not screened according to established guidelines. Although a physician is necessary to obtain semen from a sperm bank, the subsequent use of the specimen is not monitored. Clinics and individual physicians have provided clients with semen from these banks for self-insemination. Women who obtain semen for self-insemination from improperly screened donors such as relatives, friends, or social networks take unnecessary, higher risks for infection, not only with HIV but also with other sexually transmitted pathogens.

Another safety loophole is nonregulation of screening of semen donors. Screening recommendations have come from several respected sources, but physicians do not have to adhere to them. In a 1987 national survey, the Office of Technology Assessment found that only 45% of physicians practicing insemination discussed with their patients the risk of HIV infection and less than 50% tested donors for HIV antibody. However, all sperm banks canvassed did screen. The following year the screening guidelines were issued but no information has been made available on their impact on national screening practices. Until proper screening of all donors is ensured, the safety of donated semen will be compromised and recipient women will be at unnecessary risk of HIV infection.

Make Insemination Safer

Maintenance of records linking semen donors and recipients is not required, which compromises efforts to control infectious complications and raises another safety concern. The secrecy that many clients desire with regard to insemination discourages such record keeping. Donor insemination has been referred to as one of the nation's best-kept secrets. The characteristics of semen donors and the number of children each eventually sires are not monitored in the United States, thus

> *"The risk of transmitting . . . any infection during artificial insemination by donor is very low."*

leaving the process open to potential abuse. Some advocates decry this secrecy and urge the establishment of donor registries such as those that exist in Australia, New Zealand, England, and Sweden. From a public health viewpoint, records should be kept in a manner that permits notification of clients who may have been exposed to an infection or donors who may be the source without compromising the privacy of either.

Artificial insemination is safe but not completely so. How much safer it can be is not altogether clear. The lack of regulation and the ease of its use without a physician suggest that infection prevention measures should be targeted also to the consumer. An informed consumer who is aware of the risk of HIV infection and insists that the semen donor be screened in accordance with the most up-to-date recommendations will increase the safety. Physicians, women who desire pregnancy through artificial insemination by donor, and semen donors all have a role to play in preventing HIV transmission. An understanding of these roles requires that we break through the wall of secrecy that now surrounds artificial insemination by donor in the United States.

Excessive Regulation of Reproductive Technologies Would Be Unconstitutional

by John A. Robertson

About the author: *John A. Robertson is the Thomas Watt Gregory Professor at the University of Texas School of Law in Austin. A well-known expert on the topic of reproductive technology, Robertson is the author of several books, including* Children of Choice: Freedom and the New Reproductive Technologies.

Technological means of reproduction are now used by thousands of infertile couples annually to produce offspring. In the United States there are over 180 in vitro fertilization (IVF) programs that combine eggs and sperm in the laboratory and then place the resulting embryos in a woman's uterus.

IVF has also led to pregnancies in prematurely menopausal women through egg donation and has made it possible for gestational surrogates to carry children for women who can produce viable eggs but cannot carry a child to term. Thousands of children are also born each year from artificial insemination with donor sperm, which is used to compensate for male infertility or to allow women without male partners to have offspring. Finally, thousands of couples use genetic screening techniques to avoid the birth of children who have certain severe hereditary diseases.

Despite the new technologies' wide appeal to couples who are infertile or at risk for producing sick or disabled offspring, the techniques continue to generate public concern and controversy. This was evident in the intense media coverage of the first human cloning experiments, reported in the fall of 1993, and the conception and birth of twins to a woman of 60, made possible through egg donation.

Many people find the willingness of physicians to manipulate human eggs, sperm, and embryos for reproductive or genetic selection purposes to be deeply disturbing and unnatural, if not also dangerous. Some think that using surrogate

Abridged from "Liberty and Assisted Reproduction" by John A. Robertson, *Trial*, August 1994. Reprinted by permission of the author.

mothers and sperm, egg, and embryo donors to provide a couple with offspring threatens traditional conceptions of parenthood and family. Others fear that these efforts to help infertile couples will produce offspring confused about their genetic heritage or otherwise harmed psychologically because of the artificial manipulations involved in their birth. Feminist critics of these practices emphasize their potential to abuse or exploit women, since women's bodies bear the brunt of most technological means of reproduction.

The law and public policy have generally lagged behind scientific development. In the case of new reproductive technology, the law has provided little guidance for participants and has seldom specified the legal consequences of these practices.

The public often reacts strongly to reports of technological advances like the cloning of human embryos, the birth of children to older women through egg donation, and the prospect of using ovaries from aborted fetuses as a source of donor eggs. Opponents may call for a ban on some or all of these procedures because of their alleged harmful effects on embryos, offspring, families, women, and traditional concepts of parenthood and reproduction.

"Facilitative regulation, not prohibition, is the best way to ensure that new reproductive technologies achieve their intended purposes."

In France, for example, a bill outlawing egg donation to women over 50 passed the senate, and many European countries ban experiments with human embryos that would be legal in the United States.

While most U.S. jurisdictions have resisted calls to prohibit paying money to surrogates, the practice is banned in many states, and federal funding of IVF research has been restricted for many years. Few states have set up the infrastructure of rules and standards needed to provide the legal certainty about parental status that is essential if the new technologies are to be integrated successfully into society.

An important point about the legal status of reproductive technologies is that an outright ban on further research or use of a technique would be unconstitutional in most instances, for it would intrude upon or limit the basic right of individuals and couples to reproduce.

Rather than attempt to ban these procedures, public policy should aim to make sure that they are safe and effective for the people using them and that the legal status of the resulting offspring is clearly defined. Facilitative regulation, not prohibition, is the best way to ensure that new reproductive technologies achieve their intended purposes with the least social disruption.

Procreative Liberty

The close connection between traditional concepts of procreative freedom and these novel techniques is usually overlooked by opponents. Individuals or couples resort to assisted reproduction because of physical necessity. They want to satisfy the deep-seated need to have and rear biologically related offspring—a need that nature, through infertility or other barriers, has frustrated.

Infertile couples have as strong and meritorious a need to reproduce as fertile couples and should have the same right to have and rear offspring through the assistance of medical technology that fertile couples have through sexual intercourse. Because of the intimate connection between assisted reproduction techniques and procreation, a government ban on these techniques would infringe the fundamental constitutional right to procreate.

> *"A particular technology should not be banned unless it could be shown to lead to substantial, tangible harm to others."*

The right to reproduce is not explicitly stated in the U.S. Constitution. However, the Supreme Court has on many occasions recognized in dicta that procreation is among "the basic civil rights of man" and that the right to "conceive and raise one's children" is an essential one.

In *Eistenstadt v. Baird*, the Court stated: "If the right to privacy means anything, it is the right of the individual, married or single, to be free of unwarranted governmental intrusion into matters so fundamentally affecting a person as the decision whether to bear or beget a child." It follows that people should not be denied the right to procreate simply because they are infertile, any more than visually impaired people should be denied the First Amendment right to read simply because they need to use braille.

Governmental restrictions on technological treatments for infertility should have to pass the same demanding test that would apply to restrictions on coital reproduction. A particular technology should not be banned unless it could be shown to lead to substantial, tangible harm to others. Only a compelling state interest that could not be protected by less restrictive means would justify restricting an individual's or couple's efforts—whether through sexual intercourse or technological assistance—to form a family.

Nearly all the new reproductive technologies pass this test. They aim to produce healthy offspring who are biologically related to one or both of the intended rearing parents. These techniques cannot be shown to threaten the extreme harm that would justify restrictions on coital reproduction.

Criticisms

Opponents generally fear that the new techniques will harm the traditional view of family, the status of prenatal life, or the role of women—issues over which reasonable people in a pluralistic society may differ. Such differing moral or symbolic views do not justify intrusions on fundamental rights in other contexts and should not be allowed to do so when reproduction by infertile couples is at stake.

Opponents also say they seek to stop the use of technological means of reproduction in order to protect offspring from novel genetic or parenting arrangements. Yet it is hard to see how children born with the help of gamete donors or surrogates are harmed. Protecting children by preventing their birth altogether hardly benefits the children, who have no other way to be born, and whose lives, by every indication, are meaningful.

Given the deep involvement of the new techniques with procreative liberty, it would not be good public policy to attempt to ban them altogether. Society would do better to craft a set of rules that would enable interested parties to use the technology in a safe and effective way, with clear rules about parental rearing rights and duties. . . .

Infertile couples have the same right to reproduce that fertile couples have. The use of donors or surrogates is sometimes necessary to achieve that goal. Couples need certainty about future child-rearing rights and duties before they enter into donor and surrogacy arrangements. State laws that interfere with those arrangements—for example, laws that prohibit the payment of money for donated gametes or gestation or that override the parties' preconception child-rearing intentions clearly interfere with the parties' procreative liberty.

These laws should not be upheld unless their proponents can show a compelling need for interfering with the procreative liberty of infertile couples. Judged by this standard, statutes that override the preconception agreements of parties in surrogacy and gamete donation should be found unconstitutional.

> *"Infertile couples have the same right to reproduce that fertile couples have."*

In sum, the use of new reproductive technologies is intimately tied to the exercise and realization of procreative liberty—a connection that opponents of the technologies seldom acknowledge. Once this connection is seen, however, state power to go beyond facilitative regulation of these techniques is extremely limited. The best way to integrate the new reproductive technologies into the social fabric is to acknowledge the rights of infertile couples to use these methods to satisfy their reproductive needs.

Regulating Reproductive Technologies Through Court Decisions Could Harm Women

by Robert H. Blank

About the author: *Robert H. Blank is affiliated with the political science department at the University of Canterbury, New Zealand.*

Many observers who study patterns in tort law have concluded that continued expansion of tort recovery for prenatal injury is leading to the recognition of the fetus as a person. The trend toward abrogating the parental immunity rule and efforts to surmount the practical difficulties of a parent-child suit clearly presage the day when a cause of action by a child against its mother for prenatal injury might be upheld. Furthermore, criminal law has increasingly been used to constrain the choices of pregnant women or to punish them for their actions which harm the fetuses they are carrying. Although these trends are incompatible with a woman's constitutional right to abortion and threaten to contradict her procreative autonomy and bodily integrity, they demonstrate a growing legal concern for the welfare of the unborn and for a right of all children to be born with a sound mind and body.

A major influence on the way the courts, as well as the public, view the maternal-fetal relationship is technology. In fact, one issue that frames all other issues surrounding the potential conflict between the pregnant woman and the fetus centers on societal perceptions of the status of the fetus. Whether dealing with workplace hazards, coerced treatment of pregnant women, or attempts to constrain maternal behavior, the way we view the fetus is critical to our position. Rapid advances in biomedical science, as reflected in prenatal diagnosis and therapy, reproduction-aiding techniques such as in vitro fertilization, and a growing array of ever more precise genetic tests are inalterably changing our

Excerpted from "Reproductive Technology" by Robert H. Blank, *Women & Politics*, vol. 13, no. 3/4 (1993), pp. 1–17; ©1993 by The Haworth Press, Inc. Reprinted by permission of the publisher, The Haworth Press, Binghamton, N.Y.

perceptions of the fetus. In combination with a heightened understanding of fetal development and of the potentially deleterious impact of a broad range of actions of the pregnant woman, these technologies are forcing a reevaluation of maternal responsibility for fetal health. Furthermore, in a culture dominated by a fascination with technology and its ability to "fix" problems, both the public and the courts are often predisposed toward acceptance of a technology without a clear understanding of the broader implications for all the parties. . . .

The Technological Imperative and Pregnant Women

The issue of maternal responsibility for fetal health is framed by the broader social value system in the United States. Our great faith in technology and medical knowledge and over-dependence on the technological fix has not only medicalized pregnancy, but created a perfect-child mentality. This is clearly reflected in many courts' acceptance of medical "fact" in cases of forced Cesarean sections, even when "fact" is uncertain and probabilistic. Laura R. Woliver contends that reproductive technologies often contain hidden policy implications—"they increase medical intervention in women's lives, diminishing women's power over their bodies and babies." Significantly, the public's view of responsible maternal behavior is shaped by the rapidly changing technological context.

As a result of society's reliance on medical technology, when new "choices" become available to women they rapidly become obligations to make the "right" choice by "choosing" the socially approved alternative.

> The "right to choose" means very little when women are powerless . . . women make their own reproductive choices, but they do not make them just as they please; they do not make them under conditions which they themselves create but under social conditions and constraints which they, as mere individuals, are powerless to change. (Rosiland Petchesky, 1980)

Furthermore, these technologies contribute to the medicalization of reproduction which threatens the freedom and dignity of women in general. By requiring third-party involvement and dependence on medical expertise, new technologies force the woman to surrender her control over procreation. Ruth Hubbard decries the practice of making every pregnancy a medical event and sees it as a result of the economic incentives for physicians to stimulate a new need for their services during pregnancy in light of declining birth rates and increasing interest in midwifery and home birth. Barbara Katz Rothman adds that the new images of the fetus resulting from prenatal technologies are making us aware of the "unborn" as people, "but they do so at the cost of making transparent the mother." Furthermore, diagnostic technologies that pronounce judgments halfway through

"Criminal law has increasingly been used to constrain the choices of pregnant women."

177

the pregnancy make extraordinary demands on women to separate themselves from the fetus within.

> The medical status of the fetus as distinct from the woman who is pregnant is becoming a star criterion to judge a woman's behavior before, during, and after pregnancy. It is no longer only our sexuality or marital status which defines us as good woman-mothers; now, we must not smoke or drink or deny medical intervention when we are pregnant, or else we are not acting in the "best interests of the fetus." Meanwhile, obstetricians have authorized themselves to act against the wishes of the pregnant woman if necessary to "protect" the interests of the fetus. (Patricia Spallone, 1989)

Some feminists rightly argue that women bear most of the risks of any reproductive research and technological application. The history of human reproduction has been, in large measure, a story of control of women, their fertility, and fecundity by society. This control, whether self-imposed or inflicted by others in a given society, has resulted in a significant loss of freedom to women and their exclusion from many activities including intellectual creativity, waged work, and training for self-support. Women, it is alleged, have been held hostage to the reproductive needs of society throughout history. The new prenatal technologies in many ways reinforce this condition. As persons whose self-identity and social role have been defined historically in relation to their procreative capacities, then, women have a great deal at stake in questions of reproductive freedom.

> *"These technologies are forcing a reevaluation of maternal responsibility for fetal health."*

There is little doubt that the status of women is intimately related to prenatal technologies. Technology is never neutral—it both reflects and shapes social values. Because of women's critical biological role as the bearers of children, any technologies that deal with reproduction affect their social role directly. Moreover, because these technologies focus on the role of women as mothers, they could lead to diminution of other roles. Some feminists argue that too much emphasis is already placed on women as only mothers in this society. Robin Rowland insists that women must reevaluate this social overstatement of the role of motherhood. "The catchcry 'but women want it' has been sounded over and over again by the medical profession to justify continuing medical advances in this field. Women need to reevaluate just what it is they want and question this justification for turning women into living laboratories."

As Hubbard cogently states, "The point is that once such a test is available and a woman decides not to use it, if her baby is born with a disability that could have been diagnosed, it is no longer an act of fate but has become her fault." Maria Mies adds that the emphasis on quality control means for most women a loss of confidence in their own bodies and their childbearing competence. She argues that the social pressure on women to produce perfect children is already enormous today.

Despite the developing patterns in the medical and legal context of the technologies described here, it is important to understand that we can, indeed, shape the boundaries and future directions of reproductive technologies. There is a tendency upon examining the rapidity and scope of technological change to assume that its very momentum is so powerful that it denies society the capacity to manage and direct its development. Although history shows

> *"The status of women is intimately related to prenatal technologies."*

that the ability to control technology is difficult, if society so desires, significant control is possible.

Although technologies transform values and the way we think about things, the relationship between values and technology is reciprocal—values also shape the boundaries of technology. For example, surrogate motherhood became an issue in the 1980s, not because of some dramatic breakthrough in technology, but rather because of an underlying change in the way we think about reproduction. The technique for effectuating surrogate contracts as largely practiced today, donor insemination, has been in existence for over a century, but surrogacy contracts became common only in the last decade after childless couples found adoption difficult. Also contributing to the demand was a reemergence in the last decade of the importance of genetic roots and the attainment of sufficient wealth by young professionals to afford these expensive fertility interventions. Likewise, the acceptance of, or demand for, prenatal diagnosis, genetic screening, and in utero surgery is heightened by the trend toward one- or two-children families. While the "perfect child" mentality has been encouraged by advances in technology, it has also been a powerful force behind the diffusion of the technologies. This quest for the perfect child can be traced to smaller families which, in turn, reflect the changing image of the family brought on by the economic realities of raising children, a concern for population control, and drastically altered lifestyles.

Acceptable vs. Non-acceptable Uses

It is also critical to understand that medical advances can be used for many different ends and will affect different persons differently. As Michelle Stanworth notes, these technologies are controversial because they "crystallize issues at the heart of contemporary controversies over sexuality, parenthood, reproduction, and the family. . . ." The ongoing debate over these innovations should rightly focus not on whether they will continue to be developed, but rather on distinguishing acceptable from non-acceptable uses. As Michael R. Harrison states, "The technology is underway, but how we as a species choose to use it, where we allow it to be used, and when we draw limits, are critical issues for all of us, but especially for women."

Although the technologies that allow for the conscious design of children do not necessarily result in the denigration of the role of women or the mandatory invasion of their reproductive privacy, within the context of a social value system sympathetic to that end and without a conscious shaping process, the danger clearly exists. A full policy assessment of these technologies, therefore, requires close attention to their cumulative impact on women as well as to women's actual experiences as reproductive beings. Given the trends discussed here, however, those persons who firmly reject any notions of fetal interests and, thus, any constraints on pregnant women, are facing a very difficult battle against these advances in medical technology.

Moreover, growing medical evidence demonstrates that many actions by the pregnant woman can be devastating to the developing fetus. Although the U.S. Supreme Court invalidated fetal protection policies in *Automotive Workers v. Johnson Controls* (No. 89-1215, 1991), the issue of harm to the fetus through exposure to workplace hazards by either the mother or father will continue to be debated as will issues of maternal (or paternal) substance abuse and other actions that might be harmful to the fetus. These data become increasingly convincing evidence of proximate cause in prenatal injury or wrongful death torts and of negligence or even abuse in criminal cases. Unless legislatures act to protect women from liability or prosecution for alleged injury to the fetus, case law with its emphasis on the facts presented by the parties to each particular case is likely to further constrain or punish high-risk actions of pregnant women. To date, legislatures have been hesitant to take such policy initiatives, thus abdicating this responsibility to the courts.

> *"Case law . . . is likely to further constrain or punish . . . pregnant women."*

Through efforts to protect the interests of the unborn child and to deter harmful parental behavior, there is an increasing danger of compromising the autonomy and even the physical integrity of pregnant women. The rapid diffusion of these technologies and their acceptance by society is creating an environment in which the courts might be tempted to adopt very stringent standards of care for pregnant women—standards that not only dictate lifestyle choice during pregnancy, but also mandate use of prenatal diagnostic tests, genetic screening, and any other appropriate medical innovations. Although counteraction of these potent legal and medical developments in order to reshape and direct the use of these technologies is yet possible, political action must be effectively taken before these initial patterns become entrenched in the value system and legal policy.

Glossary

amniocentesis   A procedure performed during pregnancy in which a needle is inserted into the **uterus** and a sample of the fluid surrounding the **fetus** is withdrawn and analyzed to determine fetal sex or chromosomal abnormality.

ART (assisted reproductive technology)   High-tech procedures that usually include the manipulation of eggs and **sperm**.

artificial insemination   The introduction of **semen** into the **uterus** through ways other than sexual intercourse.

azoospermia   A lack of **sperm** in the **semen**.

biopsy   The removal of a sample of tissue for examination.

chorionic villus sampling (CVS)   A procedure in which fetal cells are retrieved and tested for chromosomal abnormalities.

Clomid   A fertility-enhancing drug given by injection.

cryopreservation   The process of freezing for future use; **sperm** and **embryos** are frozen and preserved through this process in many reproductive technologies.

donor insemination (DI)   The process of inseminating a woman with **sperm** obtained from a man who is not her partner.

ectopic pregnancy   A pregnancy that occurs when a fertilized egg implants outside the **uterus**, usually in one of the **fallopian tubes**; such **zygotes** cannot survive, and the pregnancy must be ended surgically because it endangers the mother's life.

embryo   The developing human from about two weeks to about eight weeks after conception.

embryo lavage   The process of washing an **embryo** out of the **uterus** for transfer or analysis.

embryo transfer   The process of moving an **embryo** created through **in vitro fertilization** to a woman's **uterus**.

endometriosis   A painful condition in which the tissue normally lining the **uterus** is found in other parts of the body, usually in the pelvic cavity.

epidural anesthesia   A form of anesthesia in which a tube is inserted into the lower spinal area to deliver drugs that numb the lower portion of the body during childbirth.

estrogen   A female sex **hormone** produced by the **ovaries** and adrenal glands that causes the development of female characteristics in women and that also plays a role in the menstrual cycle and pregnancy.

fallopian tubes   Structures located between the **uterus** and the **ovaries** that are responsible for the transport of the egg.

fertile   Capable of reproducing.

fetus   The developing human from about eight weeks' gestation until birth.

fibroid tumor   Noncancerous tumor composed of tough fibers of **uterine** muscle tissue.

follicle   Structures within the **ovary** that house immature eggs.

follicle-stimulating hormone (FSH)   A **hormone** that causes the maturation and release of one egg each month from an **ovary's follicles**.

gamete   A sex cell; that is, an egg or a **sperm**.

gamete intrafallopian transfer (GIFT)   Surgical process by which **gametes** are injected directly into a female's **fallopian tubes**.

gestational surrogate   A woman who gestates an embryo formed from the egg and **sperm** of another couple.

Glossary

hormones   Chemicals secreted by certain cells in order to specifically affect the activity of certain other cells in another part of the body.

infertile   Incapable of reproducing.

intracytoplasmic sperm injection (ICSI)   A micromanipulation technique whereby a single **sperm** is injected directly into the center of the egg.

intrauterine insemination (IUI)   Introducing **sperm** directly into the **uterus**.

in vitro fertilization (IVF)   Literally, "in glass" fertilization; fertilization outside the body in a laboratory dish; the fertilized egg is then placed in the woman's **uterus** to implant and develop normally.

in vivo   Literally, "in the living body"; refers to normal reproduction that occurs without medical assistance or intervention, as opposed to **in vitro fertilization**.

laparoscopy   Procedure in which a fiberoptic scope is inserted through the navel to view or operate on the pelvic organs; often performed to help determine possible causes of female infertility, such as obstructed **fallopian tubes**.

oocyte   An egg cell; also called an **ovum**.

ovaries   The female reproductive organs that produce eggs and hormones; human females have two ovaries.

ovum   An egg; also called an **oocyte**.

Pergonal   A fertility-enhancing drug given by injection.

semen   Male reproductive fluid composed of **sperm** and nutrient-rich fluids.

sonogram   Also called "ultrasound"; diagnostic test using sound waves to analyze internal organs; often used to study the pelvic organs to determine causes of infertility and also to determine the existence of fetal abnormalities.

sperm   The male **gamete**; when it fertilizes an egg from a female, conception occurs.

surrogate mother   A woman who conceives and bears a child for another couple, using the **sperm** of the male partner of that couple but her own egg (see also **gestational surrogate**).

Tay-Sachs disease   A genetic disease characterized by poor physical development and death by about the age of four.

uterine   Of or related to the **uterus**.

uterus   The female organ in which gestation takes place.

zona crack, dissection, and drilling   Various techniques involving the use of enzymes (biochemicals) and tiny needles to penetrate the outer membrane (zona pellucida) of the egg and permit fertilization by **sperm** during **in vitro fertilization**.

zygote   A fertilized egg that has not yet begun dividing.

zygote intrafallopian transfer (ZIFT)   Introduction directly into the **fallopian tube** of the **zygote** resulting from **in vitro fertilization**.

Bibliography

Books

Kenneth D. Alpern, ed.	*The Ethics of Reproductive Technology.* New York: Oxford University Press, 1992.
Lori B. Andrews	*Between Strangers: Surrogate Mothers, Expectant Fathers, and Brave New Babies.* New York: Harper & Row, 1989.
Susan L. Cooper and Ellen S. Glazer	*Beyond Infertility: The New Paths to Parenthood.* New York: Lexington Books, 1994.
Martha A. Field	*Surrogate Motherhood: The Legal and Human Issues.* Cambridge, MA: Harvard University Press, 1990.
Robert R. Franklin and Dorothy Brockman	*In Pursuit of Fertility.* New York: K. Holt, 1990.
Warren Freedman	*Legal Issues in Biotechnology and Human Reproduction: Artificial Conception and Modern Genetics.* Westport, CT: Quorum Books, 1991.
Herbert A. Goldfarb with Zoe Graves and Judith Greif	*Overcoming Infertility: Twelve Couples Share Their Success Stories.* New York: Wiley, 1995.
Larry Gostin, ed.	*Surrogate Motherhood: Politics and Privacy.* Bloomington: Indiana University Press, 1990.
Helen Bequaert Holmes, ed.	*Issues in Reproductive Technology: An Anthology.* New York: Garland Publishing, 1992.
Lawrence J. Kaplan and Rosemarie Tong	*Controlling Our Reproductive Destiny: A Technological and Philosophical Perspective.* Cambridge, MA: MIT Press, 1994.
Paul Lauritzen	*Pursuing Parenthood: Ethical Issues in Assisted Reproduction.* Bloomington: Indiana University Press, 1993.
Ruth Macklin	*Surrogates and Other Mothers: The Debates over Assisted Reproduction.* Philadelphia: Temple University Press, 1994.
Irina Pollard	*A Guide to Reproduction: Social Issues and Human Concerns.* New York: Cambridge University Press, 1994.
Janice G. Raymond	*Women as Wombs: Reproductive Technologies and the Battle over Women's Freedom.* San Francisco: HarperCollins, 1993.
Robyn Rowland	*Living Laboratories: Women and Reproductive Technologies.* Bloomington: Indiana University Press, 1992.
Cheryl Saban	*Miracle Child: Genetic Mother, Surrogate Womb.* Far Hills, NJ: New Horizon Press, 1993.
Bonnie Steinbock	*Life Before Birth: The Moral and Legal Status of Embryos and Fetuses.* New York: Oxford University Press, 1992.

Bibliography

| Mary Beth Whitehead with Loretta Schwartz-Nobel | *A Mother's Story: The Truth About the Baby M Case.* New York: St. Martin's Press, 1989. |

Periodicals

| Katrine Ames et al. | "And Donor Makes Three," *Newsweek*, September 30, 1991. |

| Lisa Busch | "Designer Families, Ethical Knots," *U.S. News & World Report*, May 31, 1993. |

| Susan Chira | "Of a Certain Age, and in a Family Way," *New York Times*, January 1, 1994. |

| Geoffrey Cowley | "Ethics and Embryos," *Newsweek*, June 12, 1995. |

| *Creighton Law Review* | Symposium Issue: Reproductive Rights, vol. 25, no. 5, November 1992. Available from Fred B. Rothman & Co., 10368 W. Centennial Rd., Littleton, CO 80123. |

| Donald DeMarco | "The Politicization of Motherhood," *Human Life Review*, Winter 1992. |

| Brian Doyle | "Something So Natural," *U.S. Catholic*, February 1992. |

| Diane Goldner | "Should I Donate My Eggs to Michael and Linda?" *Glamour*, January 1992. |

| *Hastings Center Report* | "What Research? Which Embryos?" January/February 1995. Available from 255 Elm Rd., Briarcliff Manor, NY 10510. |

| Ellen Hopkins | "Tales from the Baby Factory," *New York Times Magazine*, March 15, 1992. |

| Gina Kolata | "Cloning Human Embryos: Debate Erupts over Ethics," *New York Times*, October 26, 1993. |

| Gina Kolata | "Fetal Ovary Transplant Is Envisioned," *New York Times*, January 6, 1994. |

| Elizabeth Kristol | "Picture Perfect: The Politics of Prenatal Testing," *First Things*, April 1993. |

| Gina Maranto | "Delayed Childbearing," *Atlantic Monthly*, June 1995. |

| Dan Morris | "All We Wanted Was a Baby of Our Own," *U.S. Catholic*, February 1992. |

| Peggy Orenstein | "Looking for a Donor to Call Dad," *New York Times Magazine*, June 18, 1995. |

| Joseph Palca | "Doing Things with Embryos," *Hastings Center Report*, January/February 1995. |

| Barbara Katz Rothman | "The Frightening Future of Baby-Making," *Glamour*, June 1992. |

| Susan V. Seligson | "Seeds of Doubt," *Atlantic Monthly*, March 1995. |

| Larry Thompson | "Fertility with Less Fuss," *Time*, November 14, 1994. |

Organizations to Contact

The editors have compiled the following list of organizations concerned with the issues debated in this book. The descriptions are derived from materials provided by the organizations. All have publications or information available for interested readers. The list was compiled on the date of publication of the present volume; names, addresses, and phone numbers may change. Be aware that many organizations take several weeks or longer to respond to inquiries, so allow as much time as possible.

The American Fertility Society
1209 Montgomery Hwy.
Birmingham, AL 35216-2809
(205) 978-5000
fax: (205) 978-5005

The society is composed of more than ten thousand physicians and scientists interested in studying fertility in humans and animals and in researching and treating infertility. It has listings of infertility specialists and clinics and offers numerous publications on the ethics of reproductive technologies and success rate of specific procedures. The society also publishes the monthly journal *Fertility and Sterility* and the quarterly newsletter *Fertility News*.

American Life League (ALL)
PO Box 1350
Stafford, VA 22555
(703) 659-4171
fax: (703) 659-2586

ALL is an educational pro-life organization that opposes abortion, artificial contraception, reproductive technologies, and fetal experimentation. It asserts that it is immoral to perform experiments on living human embryos and fetuses, whether inside or outside of the mother's womb. ALL further contends that surrogate motherhood is contrary to moral law and violates the sanctity of marriage. Its publications include the policy statement *Creating a Pro-Life America*, the paper *What Is Norplant?* and the booklets *Medical Ethics: Its Accommodation of Abortion and the Effects* and *Contraceptive Compromise: The Perfect Crime*.

Center for Biomedical Ethics
Box 33 UMHC
Minneapolis, MN 55455
(612) 625-4917

The center seeks to advance and disseminate knowledge concerning ethical issues in health care and the life sciences. It conducts original research, offers educational programs, fosters public discussion and debate, and assists in the formulation of public policy. The center publishes a quarterly newsletter and reading packets on specific topics, including fetal tissue research.

Center for Surrogate Parenting
8383 Wilshire Blvd., Suite 750
Beverly Hills, CA 90211

(213) 655-1974
fax: (213) 852-1310

The center disseminates information on the legal, moral, ethical, and psychological aspects of surrogate parenting. It publishes a newsletter on new procedures, events, and statistics concerning surrogacy. The center also publishes the semiannual newsletter *Center for Surrogate Parenting*.

The Couple to Couple League (CCL)
PO Box 111184
Cincinnati, OH 45211
(513) 661-7612

CCL promotes natural family planning, a method that relies on a woman's natural fertility cycle. The organization believes that natural birth-control practices are healthier and more morally acceptable than the use of artificial contraceptives that are considered abortifacient. CCL has numerous publications on the topic, including the books *The Medical Hazards of the Birth Control Pill*, *Abortion: Questions and Answers*, and *The Bible and Birth Control* and the brochures *The Effectiveness of Natural Family Planning* and *The Pill and IUD: Some Facts for an Informed Choice*.

Fertility Research Foundation
877 Park Ave.
New York, NY 10021
(212) 744-5500
fax: (212) 744-6536

The foundation provides therapeutic, diagnostic, and consultational services for childless couples. It conducts a wide array of infertility studies and maintains research projects on human reproduction. Although it has no regular publications, the foundation has information for the public concerning human reproduction and infertility.

Hastings Center
255 Elm Rd.
Briarcliff Manor, NY 10510
(914) 762-8500

Since its founding in 1969, the Hastings Center has played a pivotal role in exploring the medical, ethical, and social ramifications of biomedical advances such as the new reproductive technologies. The center publishes books, papers, guidelines, and the bimonthly *Hastings Center Report*.

Institute for Reproductive Health
433 S. Beverly Dr.
Beverly Hills, CA 90212
(310) 553-5821
(800) 562-4426
fax: (213) 854-4549

The institute works to educate women about their rights and responsibilities concerning their reproductive health. It conducts research and disseminates information on issues such as reproductive technologies, female reconstructive surgery, sexually transmitted diseases, hysterectomy, and surgical abuses against women. It publishes *Women's Health Quarterly*.

National Association of Surrogate Mothers (NASM)
8383 Wilshire Blvd., Suite 750
Beverly Hills, CA 90211
(213) 655-2015
fax: (213) 852-1310

The association supports surrogacy and seeks to educate the public concerning surrogate mothers. It lobbies for legislation to regulate the surrogate-mother industry and to protect and define the legal rights of surrogate mothers. The association publishes the quarterly *NASM Newsletter*.

National Women's Health Network
1325 G St. NW
Washington, DC 20003
(202) 347-1140

The network studies and provides information to the public on all aspects of women's health, including reproductive issues. Its periodic newsletter provides information on reproductive technologies.

Organization of Parenting Through Surrogacy (OPTS)
750 N. Fairview St.
Burbank, CA 91505
(818) 848-3761

A national network, OPTS promotes the concept of parenthood through surrogate mothers. It offers information and lobbies legislatures to pass laws in support of surrogacy. OPTS publishes a periodic newsletter and maintains a listing of surrogate/parenting centers.

Resolve, Inc.
1310 Broadway
Somerville, MA 02244-1731
(617) 623-1156
fax: (617) 623-0252

Founded in 1977, Resolve is a national organization dedicated to serving the needs of people dealing with infertility. It has a national office and local chapters that provide information on numerous topics concerning infertility. Resolve publishes the quarterly *Resolve National Newsletter*.

Index